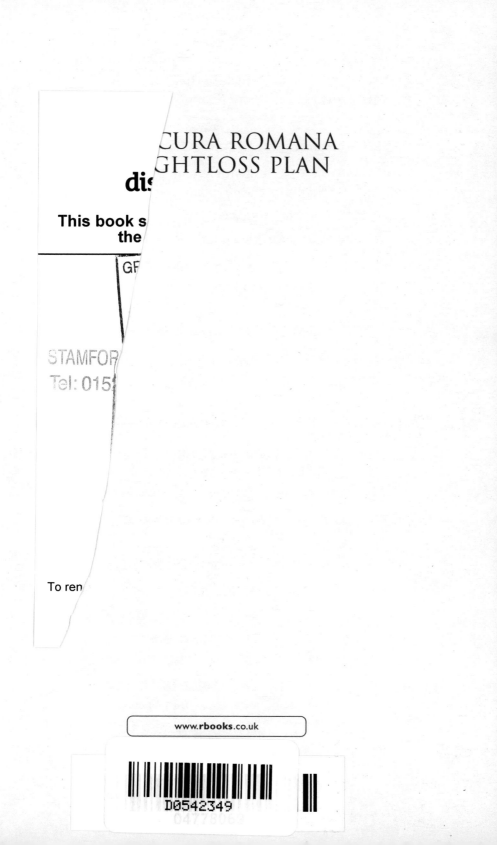

CURA ROMANA
GHTLOSS PLAN

dis

This book s
the

GF

To ren

THE CURA ROMANA WEIGHTLOSS PLAN

Transform Your Looks, Energy and Life, Now and Long Into the Future

Leslie Kenton

BANTAM PRESS

LONDON · TORONTO · SYDNEY · AUCKLAND · JOHANNESBURG

TRANSWORLD PUBLISHERS
61–63 Uxbridge Road, London W5 5SA
A Random House Group Company
www.randomhouse.co.uk

First published in Great Britain
in 2011 by Bantam Press
an imprint of Transworld Publishers

A CIP catalogue record for this book
is available from the British Library.

ISBN 9780593066737

Addresses for Random House Group Ltd companies outside the UK
can be found at: www.randomhouse.co.uk
The Random House Group Ltd Reg. No. 954009

The Random House Group Limited supports The Forest Stewardship
Council (FSC®), the leading international forest certification organisation.
Our books carrying the FSC label are printed on FSC® certified paper.
FSC is the only forest certification scheme endorsed by the leading environmental
organisations, including Greenpeace. Our paper procurement policy can be found at
www.randomhouse.co.uk/environment

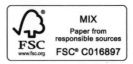

Typeset in 11/15pt Celeste by
Falcon Oast Graphic Art Ltd.
Printed and bound in Great Britain by
Clays Ltd, Bungay, Suffolk

2 4 6 8 10 9 7 5 3

CONTENTS

AUTHOR'S NOTE

Welcome to Leslie Kenton's Cura Romana®, a unique weightloss and well-being programme which will not only take you on a journey of transformation and discovery, but will enhance your life emotionally, physically and spiritually.

Based on a weightloss plan devised more than half a century ago, Leslie Kenton's Cura Romana® has been created for men and women who want to lose more than 6 pounds and who want to leave behind, once and for all, the struggles with their weight. It is not recommended for those wishing to lose less than this or for pregnant women or nursing mothers. Before embarking on this or any weightloss programme, you should consult your medical practitioner. This is particularly important if you are taking medication, since the improvement in health is often so dramatic that your doctor will need to monitor the levels of medication you are on, reducing it as he or she finds necessary.

Following years of research and mentoring, I am delighted to be able to guide you through this special experience, step by step. If at any time you feel in need of further advice, information or support, please visit the Cura Romana website: *www.curaromana.com.*

For those who do not have issues with their weight, but who wish to experience the health- and life-enhancing benefits the Cura Romana programme offers – or indeed for those who have experienced the benefits of this programme and want to continue on their journey of freedom and transformation – it is my hope and my dream that an advanced development of Cura Romana for these purposes will be launched in the near future. Many life-enhancing gifts from carefully formulated homeopathic hCG combined with A. T. W. Simeons' work await our discovery.

I wish you health and happiness.

Leslie Kenton

The material in this book is intended for information purposes only. None of the suggestions or information is meant in any way to be prescriptive. Any attempt to treat a medical condition should always come under the direction of a competent physician. Neither the publisher nor I can accept responsibility for injuries or illness arising from failure by a reader to take medical advice.

I am only a reporter, but one who has researched, broadcast and written about obesity, natural health and A. T. W. Simeons' work for forty years. I have always had a profound interest in helping myself and others to maximize our potential for well-being of body, mind and spirit so we are able to live at a high level of energy, consciousness and creativity.

FOREWORD

Leon I. Hammer, MD

'**D**OES CURA ROMANA WORK?' Naturally this is any reader's primary concern. Let me begin by describing my own experience on the Protocol, and that of my wife. A year ago, Leslie Kenton offered us the opportunity of being guided through the Cura Romana programme.

The day we began, my wife, aged sixty-eight, weighed 139 pounds. All her adult life she had been dissatisfied with the shape of her body, especially her legs. She lost 19 pounds. Now, a year later, she has effortlessly sustained her weightloss within a pound of what it was at the end of the programme. She now has the body shape she had dreamed of since she was a girl and she is free of the food cravings that had plagued her since childhood. She has also experienced a reduction in the frequency and severity of migraine headaches which she has suffered since the age of eleven. Her headaches used to require trips to the emergency room, where intra-muscular Demerol (a synthetic narcotic) with Compazine (an anti-nausea medication) had to be administered. In the past year she has had only one or two migraines (instead of the one to three a week which she had been having). Both responded immediately to aspirin or Excedrin-Migraine.

Before I began the Protocol I had for months been experiencing severe backache. It did not respond to acupuncture, herbs or massage.

A few hours after I took my first dose of hCG the pain was gone. It has not returned.

I was eighty-five years old when we began the programme and I weighed 144 pounds. I had a moderate 'beer belly' – as I told Leslie – without the benefit of beer. The beer belly disappeared and my weight steadily reduced. Now, at age eighty-six, my weight remains between 128 and 131 pounds. I feel lighter. I kayak regularly and play tennis twice a week with a partner half my age.

As created by A. T. W. Simeons, then further developed and perfected by Leslie Kenton, Cura Romana does indeed *work*. It requires only three weeks of careful monitoring of food eaten, followed by six weeks of Consolidation. Neither my wife nor I was ever hungry on 500 calories a day. During Consolidation, she and I became aware of the foods that did not make each of us feel good. We learned this by gradually introducing and testing them to find out which foods our bodies handled well and which they did not. Now, we automatically avoid the latter.

While success is the ultimate practical test of any theory, the process by which success is achieved is most important to those of us who, like Simeons, Kenton and myself, know that the enduring benefit of any achievement depends upon having identified the root cause, which is being addressed.

When I attended a 'scientific' high school in the late 1930s, a debate began between a friend and myself about cancer. Subsequently we both became physicians, so the debate continued. He was convinced that cancer would be 'cured' in a few years. His conviction was based on the vast escalation of pharmaceuticals after World War II. He believed, as many did at that time, that they were revolutionizing medicine.

I argued that, since cancer was a mutation of the cell's chromosomes, the answer to it would need to be found through an in-depth understanding of genetics and of that which creates, arrests and reverses mutations. This difference in scientific philosophy eventually led to our disaffection.

In the ensuing seventy years it has been evident that my friend's approach has not worked. And, although a knowledge base in genetics has grown significantly, this has not had the financial backing of the pharmaceutical industry or government to make it possible for extensive genetic cancer research to be carried out. The root cause of cancer remains undiscovered.

Not so for Simeons and Kenton. Simeons' success with hCG and Fröhlich's syndrome stirred his curiosity. (Einstein said, 'I have no special talents. I am only passionately curious.') Simeons' awareness of the need to identify the root cause in disturbed regulation of fat metabolism – the ultimate quest for the holy grail of obesity – led to his having located the locus of the issue in the diencephalon: the thalamus, hypothalamus and pituitary.

He chose to ignore the prevailing medical model of 'evidence-based medicine', the validity of which is built on a statistical-mathematical, deductive, digital-linear model in which one begins with an assumption, then limits observations to the paradigms within which this notion has been constructed. Instead, Simeons employed inductive-logic and experience-based medicine in which one builds a theory from observations – a method which has long been the basis of successful indigenous medicines, such as Chinese, Tibetan and Ayurvedic, all of which are still vitally extant in our time.

Kenton observes that 'Simeons was a master of observation and practicality. He refused to be side-tracked by facile beliefs about obesity.' Kenton quotes my personal medical mentor, Claude Bernard, as saying that to have an idea about a natural phenomenon, we must first of all observe it. All human knowledge is limited to working back from observed effects to their cause. The ongoing attempt from 'evidence-based medical research' to eliminate all inductive-based medicine, wisdom and bodies of knowledge continues to this day. As Kenton states with regard to Simeons' methodology, 'If anything, the furore rages even more vehemently now than it ever has'.

In my own practice, I have persistently urged the medical community to abhor the trend of our times for seeking immediate gratification by treating symptoms instead of searching for the root of medical conundrums, as Simeons and Kenton have done.

As Kenton cogently illustrates, and as Simeons himself appreciated, the root cause for obesity may lie even deeper than the diencephalon – including within it the relationship between insulin, hCG and leptin, for instance, which has yet to be elucidated. There may be many other factors as well which have yet to be identified.

In this book, Kenton has moved Simeons' work in a new direction by making these remarkable discoveries available to a great many people rather than only to those economically fortunate enough to afford to partake of it in clinics. By following the thread from the injectable to the oral, and finally to the homeopathic, she has engaged knowledgeable experts to assist her in developing the practical Protocol with which this book is concerned.

Finally, I must add a word about this remarkable woman. Leslie Kenton, whom I have known for almost forty years, has tirelessly reconstructed her own life from the detritus of her childhood – as recorded in her recent book *Love Affair* – for which she takes full responsibility. Thanks to her ability to think 'outside the box' while adhering to impeccable standards of research and trial, she has turned her own physical trauma and pain, as well as the subsequent immobility and weight gain, not only into an effective quest for the truth about obesity but beyond, sharing knowledge about health and life which encompasses more profound aspects of our existence. She has helped herself and others to make deep connections with their own essential being. It was she who, in 1971, introduced me – with my orthodox medical and psychiatric background – to Chinese medicine. In 2009 she restored my wife and myself with the gift of our bodies' true weight, shape and functioning. I have no doubt that in the future there will be many more gifts for all of us coming from this fertile, inquiring soul.

Leon I. Hammer, MD

PREFACE

IF SOMEONE TOLD YOU that you could shed your excess fat, create high-level health and transform the way you feel about yourself and your life in nine weeks, what would you say? I know what I would have said: 'Absurd – impossible – what nonsense!' That was before I discovered homeopathic Cura Romana – before I experienced for myself the transformation it brings physically, emotionally and spiritually.

I had long been familiar with the *original* Cura Romana protocol, developed in Rome by a far-sighted British physician more than half a century ago. I had proved to myself its unique ability to bring about safe, rapid weightloss without hunger – an impressive feat in its own right. I knew even then that I had stumbled upon something really important – a life-altering discovery – and I wanted to tell everyone about it. But the original Cura Romana was a *medical* programme. It was available only at a few expensive clinics in the world. It could be given only under strict supervision by a doctor highly trained in the method.

Like a racehorse at the gate, I kept champing at the bit, longing to share my findings – to write about Cura Romana in an article or a book. But how could I write about something available only to a privileged few when there were such vast numbers of overweight people who could never experience it? Cura Romana was meant to belong to everyone. I was sure of this. So I remained silent – vowing I would not write or publicly speak about Cura Romana until, through some serendipitous event, it could be made available in a non-medical form to *everyone*. Three years ago, this became possible.

This book tells the story of how Leslie Kenton's Cura Romana® came into being. It speaks of the genius physician who created the most powerful and effective treatment for obesity in the world. It explores how this Protocol restores balanced functioning to the body's appetite- and weight-control centre in the brain and how it brings an end to cravings and compulsive eating. It reports on the experience of doctors who have long used it. It shares personal experiences from hundreds of people whom I have mentored on their Cura Romana Journeys, men and women from Britain and the United States, Africa, South America, Europe, Oceania and the Middle East. Most important of all, this book presents the inside story. It gives you the nuts and bolts of Cura Romana. It tells how you can experience its blessings for yourself should you wish to bring an end to your own struggles with overweight.

My writing this book has been the fulfilment of a dream I've nurtured for more than two decades – that of sharing the Cura Romana experience with others who, like myself, have longed for a lasting solution to weight problems yet doubted they would ever find one.

May your frustration, disappointment and self-criticism come to an end. And may you – whoever and wherever you are – come to live your life out of your magnificent essential self in the process.

Leslie Kenton

PART ONE

THE
DISCOVERY

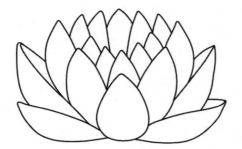

My Story

A BAVARIAN DOCTOR and friend – the world's most respected authority on *live cell therapy* – first introduced me to Cura Romana twenty years ago. One day, while visiting his clinic, I mentioned to him that since adolescence I had struggled with my weight. He smiled.

'How much do you know about Cura Romana?' he asked.

'Cura what?'

'Cura Romana – the Roman Cure.'

'Nothing,' I replied. 'What is it?'

Instead of telling me, he handed me a book written and privately published more than half a century ago by a British doctor – A. T. W. Simeons.

'Read this,' he said.

I read the book in less than two hours. I was fascinated. It was obvious that the physician who wrote it was highly intelligent and a deep thinker. He had a profound understanding of how the body works in all its complexities, including the all-encompassing interconnections between body and psyche.

Having spent many years ploughing through stilted scientific medical papers for my work in health, I found the straightforward, clear way in which he wrote refreshing. There was none of the usual pompous hedge-your-bets stuff you find in books and medical papers written by most scientists and doctors. The only trouble I had while reading it was that – having struggled with my own weight for so long – I hardly dared to believe that the information it contained could be real. If Cura Romana delivered its promises, for me it would be a dream come true.

'He claims to have discovered the cause and cure for obesity,' I said to my doctor friend. 'I find that hard to believe.'

'Why not try it? Find out for yourself,' he replied, smiling.

He knew me well. He knew that I never take anything on faith, no matter how many so-called 'experts' tell me I should. I need to experience something first hand. I have to *know* it from within.

Proof of the Pudding

Disbelieving and apprehensive, yet determined to find out if what Simeons had written was true, every morning I showed up at the nurse's office. She weighed me, then injected me with 125 International Units (IUs) of a natural substance called *human chorionic gonadotrophin* (hCG), which you will learn all about soon. She gave me a diet sheet setting out what foods I could and couldn't eat and told me exactly how much of each I was allowed. She said I must stop using my face creams and body lotions, explaining that any animal or vegetable fats or oils they contained would be absorbed through the skin and would interfere with weightloss. Meanwhile, my doctor friend forbade me to go for my morning run. This was the one thing I loved doing each day and which I then believed was keeping my body reasonably lean.

'You don't need it,' he said. 'Let the Protocol do its job and just trust the process.'

Food for Life

HCG is a natural substance secreted in a woman's body during pregnancy. Its purpose is to make sure that the foetus has adequate nourishment even in times of famine. HCG liberates fat deposits from a pregnant woman's long-term fat stores and turns them into a source of food for the developing baby. Used for weightloss on Cura Romana, this substance triggers the hypothalamus gland in the brain, enabling the body to burn up fat from long-term fat stores, transforming it into energy for living. This means that, even while you are asleep and dreaming blissfully, your body goes on burning fat.

I had never been anywhere *near* as slim as I wanted to be – at least not since I was thirteen. At that time I'd been subjected to what is euphemistically known as *electro-convulsive therapy* (ECT). This was an unsuccessful attempt to wipe out memories of severe traumas experienced while growing up. The ECT damaged parts of my brain. From that moment onwards I could no longer remember telephone numbers or solve complex mathematical problems. It also screwed up my metabolism and rendered me hypothyroid – something which my doctor discovered a year or so later. Apparently the brain damage from the ECT had triggered my body to begin laying down unwanted fat. When, at the age of nineteen, I went to work as a Ford model in New York, Eileen Ford insisted I shed 20 pounds. I succeeded in doing this only through a determined act of will. I stopped eating.

During each of my pregnancies (I have four children) I gained masses of weight – between 40 and 60 pounds. Like many women, I had followed the nonsensical dictate that you need to 'eat for two'. Afterwards, thanks to having breastfed each of my children, and to my growing knowledge about health, not to mention the passion I had developed for exercise and eating a high-raw diet, I would lose what I had gained after the birth. But it was always a monumental struggle. And despite my love of running – and later of weight training – that struggle would go on for more than thirty years.

A stunning experience

Back to Bavaria. After one week on the Cura Romana Protocol, living on a measly 500 calories a day – protein foods like beef, fish and chicken, plus green vegetables and a couple of pieces of fruit each day – I had lost 10 pounds. I'd experienced no hunger. I had energy to spare. I was sleeping as deeply and peacefully as a child, yet seemed to need only six hours a night. I would wake each morning full of excitement about the day ahead. I couldn't remember ever having felt so good.

Want to hear more? My skin glowed. When I looked in the mirror I witnessed the true shape of my face emerging. I realized that my bone structure had long been covered over by puffiness. By the end of three weeks, my weightloss was somewhere between 15 and 18 pounds – I no longer remember exactly. Even more surprising, the fat had come off from all the *right* places, like my legs and waist. This was fat I had never been able to get rid of no matter how much I'd tried. I could see that the natural size and shape of my body was coming to birth.

The Quest Begins

I love research. I think this comes from being born with an obsession to dig deeper and deeper in an attempt to penetrate and come to understand any mystery that fascinates me. Determined to learn as much as I could, layer by layer I began to uncover the Cura Romana story. I found reports filled with celebration and triumph, and clinical studies validating Simeons' claims. I also came upon tales told by idiots, 'full of sound and fury, signifying nothing', including deliberately distorted – occasionally bizarre – research discrediting the Protocol.

Since A. T. W. Simeons' death in 1970, the Roman Cure has continued to change the lives of men and women able to afford treatment at a few reputable clinics in Europe, South America and – to some extent – the United States. For, when Simeons published his first paper on the Roman Cure in the mid-1950s, doctors from around the world flocked to Rome to be trained in the Protocol, then returned to their own countries to make use of what they had learned.

I also discovered that not everyone claiming to offer Simeons' 'hCG diet' knew what they were doing. Many did not even appear to care. Fly-by-night fat farms of dubious quality sprang up in the 1960s, run by practitioners more interested in money-making than in helping people end their struggles with obesity. Weightloss has always been a lucrative business. Like the proverbial snake-oil salesmen who once travelled the American byways selling their 'cure-alls', the fly-by-nighters wanted their own piece of the action.

Big Pharma Wakes Up

HCG is a generic substance of natural origin. It is therefore not *patentable*. Pharmaceutical corporations make billions each year selling their patented drugs. With all the fuss Simeons' Protocol had generated, drug companies came to see it as a threat. They still do. If Cura Romana were shown to keep its promises, at best this would be a thorn in their sides. At worst it would result in an enormous loss of revenue.

The sale of weightloss drugs and over-the-counter products has always been dependent on people going on diets, losing some weight and then regaining it. Statistically, more than 90 per cent of people on weightloss diets do this. That is what keeps them flocking back to buy more drugs. Cura Romana had created such a huge buzz in the medical community and among people who had experienced Simeons' treatment that its success drew the attention of the Food and Drug Administration (FDA) in the United States.

The FDA is not an agency dedicated to improving human health. It is an organization serving the financial interests of the pharmaceutical industry. So much is this the case that negative attention from the FDA often tells you that the reported health benefits from a product or treatment are significant enough to undermine drug profits. After publication of a few negative research trials – virtually all too small or badly designed and poorly implemented to be taken seriously – the FDA declared that 'hCG is of no use for obesity management' on the grounds that 'similar results can be experienced with or without the hCG by following a very low calorie diet.'

The Europe connection

While this was going on in the New World, across the waters in Germany, Holland, Italy, Austria and Switzerland practitioners trained in Simeons' method – including endocrinologists, plastic surgeons and university professors – went on successfully treating their patients with Cura Romana. They knew from their own clinical experience that the Protocol delivered reliable, fast, safe, hunger-free weightloss. As Simeons himself said, 'The protocol works for everybody so long as it is followed exactly'. Some of these physicians and surgeons would go on to do their own research projects and publish their results.

From the mid-1970s onwards, Cura Romana went underground, but more about this in 'The Drama' (see page 49). Then in 2007 an event changed all this. A book was published in the United States about the 'hCG diet'. Although the book grossly distorts Simeons' Protocol, its arrival on the scene triggered another epidemic of hCG fever. It also fuelled the dissemination of a lot of false information about the diet and created havoc. YouTube filled up with videos shot by amateur enthusiasts who had ordered injectable hCG from drug companies outside the United States and recorded their own do-it-yourself experiences – trials, tribulations, successes and failures. Other videos offered demonstrations of how to inject yourself or take hCG orally.

In the wake of all this hullabaloo, spas and health practitioners in the United States began to invent their own protocols to go with the sale of hCG. Many involved money-spinning 'extra products' people were being urged to buy. The profiteers then boasted – inaccurately – that everyone loses between 1 and 2 pounds a day on their programmes. Amidst subsequent confusion, misinformation and profiteering, and despite the way the book distorted Simeons' original Protocol, the book's publication did something genuinely valuable: it brought to public awareness the fact that Simeons' work existed and it made his privately published book *Pounds and Inches* available as a free download on dozens of websites.

Crippling Accidents

About the time all this was taking place, I was recovering from four serious accidents. They had resulted in severe pain in my lower body, making me unable to exercise. For eighteen months I was not even able to walk more than a few yards. This had plunged me into a despondent state and led me to retreat inside a walled garden, where I wrote a memoir about my childhood and my family – *Love Affair*. The writing of this book, which was the most challenging thing I had ever written, took me to the depths of my soul. In the process and, in no small part, as a result of the injuries and immobility, I had gained a lot of weight. When I finished writing the book, I was determined to lose the weight I'd gained and restore the use of my legs. How? This I knew for certain. I would return to Cura Romana.

Transformation begins

I rang my doctor friend in Bavaria. He sent the ampoules of hCG I would need and I began the Protocol, injecting myself with 125 IU of hCG each morning. I lost weight steadily and with ease. Once again, Cura Romana was clearing away the distortions in the size and shape of my body that had developed during this difficult period. And my passion to celebrate Simeons' work and make it available to a wider public became stronger than ever.

I searched the internet to find out who was working with Simeons' Protocol, and where and how. I resurrected a connection I had made years before with a much-respected Argentinian doctor who, having worked in Europe with a Swiss plastic surgeon for more than twenty years, had developed a well-tested oral form of hCG to be used on the Protocol. I contacted an obstetrician and gynaecologist in Vienna, an endocrinologist in Germany, an American MD in Arizona, a surgeon in Spain and others who were still using Cura Romana with integrity.

I came across a handful of doctors and naturopaths who had abandoned the use of both injectable and oral hCG in its drug form in favour of a homeopathic remedy made from it. My reaction to learning this was almost identical to what it had been when my Bavarian doctor friend introduced me to the injectable Protocol all those years before: '*Homeopathic* hCG? Surely that can't work. You've got to use the *real thing*.' These men and women insisted that they got the same results for weightloss with the homeopathic as they did with the injectable.

I had to find out for myself if this was true. I ordered two bottles of an American-made homeopathic to experiment with. They arrived in the post smack in the middle of my weightloss programme on which, until that day, I had been using the injections. I stopped the injections immediately. The next day I began putting drops of the homeopathic under my tongue a few times a day and waited to see what would happen. Nothing was altered. My excess fat continued to fall away exactly as it had been doing on the injectable. A few weeks later I had shed all the weight I intended to lose.

A shared dream

With every week that passed on Cura Romana, I felt stronger and better than I had for years. I shared all this with my youngest son, Aaron. I began to work with other people who were keen to experience in their own lives the transformation they had witnessed in me. Aaron was intrigued by what he saw happening. The more he and I talked about it, the more sure we became that the best way to reach vast numbers of people who could benefit from the Cura Romana experience was for us to put together a website. There was only one problem. We had no idea how to go about this. What had long been my dream became a dream that Aaron and I had come to share.

Like two people who had never built a house, we were forced to start from the ground up. All we knew was this was something we intended to do, that we wanted to do it together and we wanted to do it all by ourselves. Aaron, with his background in film-making and design, set about learning the technical skills he needed to create a website that would be both beautiful and functional. I continued mentoring a rapidly growing number of people privately. I wanted to explore how the Protocol works with men and women of all sizes and ages and to hone my mentoring skills. The more I did, the more passionate the two of us became. We were continually surprised by the extent of the transformations homeopathic Cura Romana brought to bodies, health and lives.

Hiccups and all – a few months later Leslie Kenton's Cura Romana® went live. The two of us found ourselves working with all sorts of people from around the world. My years of waiting and hoping that Cura Romana could one day be available to everyone in a non-medical form had come to an end. I woke up one morning to the realization that *www.curaromana.com* had turned our dreams into a living reality. And I smiled.

THE ROMAN CURE

IT'S TIME to lay aside for a while everything you know – or think you know – about weightloss. Why? Because the Roman Cure is like nothing else in the world. Its goal is not just to help your body shed unwanted fat rapidly. Its aim is to re-balance the centre of appetite control and fat-burning in the brain, thereby restoring healthy metabolic processes. So, once you have finished the rapid weightloss part of the programme, your body is able to burn calories from the foods you eat in the way it is designed to do and to turn them into energy instead of laying them down as fat stores.

Despite what we're constantly told in the media, neither regular exercise nor eating good food prevents weight gain. Nor can they bring about permanent weightloss *unless* this fat-control centre is functioning correctly. In those of us who continually struggle with our weight, this important part of the brain is not working as it should.

The Reset

Cura Romana relies equally on two key factors to accomplish its metabolic reset. The first is an *exacting*, very low-calorie diet. The second is a specific homeopathic made from hCG. Together they spur fat-burning, enabling your body to shed between half a pound and a pound a day – safely, with little or no hunger. These two powerhouses depend on each other to work their magic. The homeopathic on its own will do nothing for weightloss. The diet on its own would be potentially dangerous. It would burn up muscle tissue as well as fat and leave you energetically depleted, with sagging skin to boot. Don't ever try it.

Collaboration

It took more than two years for me and John Morgan, a qualified pharmacist, to develop the homeopathic we use on Leslie Kenton's Cura Romana®. We created it using the only natural substance known to man capable of directing the body to turn unwanted fat stores into usable energy – hCG. (For information on how to obtain the homeopathic spray, see 'Resources', page 340).

John's background and introduction to homeopathy are interesting. In the 1970s he was working in a pharmacy and, having witnessed the downward spiral that some people get into when treated with drugs, he had begun to question their effectiveness. He started to explore other possibilities. 'It may sound odd,' he says, 'but the thing that really changed the way I viewed it all was my working in a pharmacy next door to a fruit and vegetable shop. One day it occurred to me that the fruit and vegetable shop was probably doing more good for its customers than I was.' He looked into homeopathy, discovered he had a knack for formulas, spent three more years studying at the College of Homeopathy in London and never looked back.

'Making homeopathic medicines is incredibly satisfying,' he says. 'Pharmacists today do very little preparation of medicines. They don't even have to count the pills out. When we make a homeopathic remedy we use a pestle and mortar to grind up a herb or other substance. I must be one of the few pharmacists using the skills we were taught in college.'

What is Homeopathy?

Homeopathy is a medical science dating back more than 200 years.

In 1796, Samuel Hahnemann published his 'Essay on a New Curative Principle', a treatise in which he established the principles of what is now known as classical homeopathy. Hahnemann (1755–1843) was a German physician, well known for his work in chemistry, pharmacology and toxicology. He theorized that a substance that can create symptoms in a healthy person could be used in smaller doses to cure those symptoms during illness. This proved to be true and became one of the fundamental tenets of homeopathy.

Homeopathy relies on minute doses of specially prepared natural substances, stimulating the body to improve its functioning. Homeopathic remedies are gentle enough to use on infants, the elderly and pets, yet potent enough to create quick and often lasting relief from abnormal functioning. Homeopathy is frequently referred to as 'energy medicine'. This is because the original substance from which a homeopathic is made can be subjected to so many physical dilutions that – in higher potencies – none of the original physical substance remains. Only a highly energetic molecular imprint of the original material is present.

In the past forty years, new approaches to homeopathy have developed. Combination homeopathy is one of them. It combines ingredients and/or potencies for its results – relying on the body's innate biological wisdom to make use of the particular potency or frequency that it requires. It's a bit like a radio tuner that can pick up the specific frequency appropriate for the station required while ignoring the rest.

Energy from Fat Stores

Testing out our homeopathic remedies, with the help of participants who worked closely with me during their own Cura Romana Journeys, was fascinating. After a year and a half, John and I settled on the right combination of hCG potencies and the Leslie Kenton's Cura Romana® formula that we now use came into being.

The homeopathic, together with the very specific dietary Protocol, burns fat stores at somewhere between 1,500 and 4,000 calories a day, turning them into pure energy.

> **Simeons says:** *Just as the daily dose of hCG is the same in all cases, so the same diet proves to be satisfactory for a small elderly lady of leisure or a hard-working muscular giant. Under the effect of hCG the obese body is always able to obtain all the calories it needs from the abnormal fat deposits, regardless of whether it uses up 1500 or 4000 per day. It must be made very clear to the patient that he is living to a far greater extent on the fat which he is losing than on what he eats.*

This means that on the programme you live more on energy generated from the fat-burning taking place in your body than on calories from the foods you eat. This is the most important thing for you to understand about how the programme works. It is also the reason that people on the programme experience little or no hunger. By now more than 200,000 people around the world have experienced the gifts of Cura Romana and come to sing its praises.

Here are a few of the benefits reported by men and women I have personally mentored on the programme:

- a need for less sleep
- an end to addictions
- an end to emotional eating

- an end to food cravings
- an end to unnatural hunger
- appetite normalized
- better hormonal balance
- better-quality sleep
- better skin
- blood pressure normalized
- blood sugar stabilized
- excellent emotional balance
- excellent loss of fat deposits on 'problem areas' such as hips, bellies and thighs
- heightened self-esteem
- improved body shape
- improved metabolism
- increased vitality
- lessening or disappearance of aches and pains
- lessening or disappearance of menopausal symptoms
- lessening or disappearance of menstrual problems
- life transformation

In the next few chapters we'll look at how Cura Romana came into being. We'll also delve into its technical aspects. For now, let's take a quick peek at the diet itself.

The nine-week Protocol is divided into two parts:

1 hCG+Food Plan, which consists of taking the hCG spray plus a strictly controlled food allowance. This is the rapid weightloss section of the programme – which lasts for exactly twenty-four days.

2 Consolidation follows and lasts for six weeks. During this part of the programme the metabolic reset is literally *consolidated* for lasting weightloss and enhanced physical and emotional well-being.

See the following At-a-Glance Guide to the Cura Romana Weightloss Plan, which will act as a useful reminder of what you're aiming to achieve and how.

At-a-Glance Guide to Leslie Kenton's Cura Romana® Weightloss Plan

Days 1 and 2: Feast Days

During these two days you will use your spray four times each day and, at the same time, eat your fill of starches and fats in preparation for impending weightloss.

These Feast Days build up the stores of glycogen and essential fats so that the body's transition into fat-burning takes place as gently as possible.

It takes 2–3 days of using the homeopathic remedy for excess fat to begin circulating in the bloodstream so it can become available in the form of usable life energy.

First 3 Weeks (Days 3–24): hCG+Food Plan

During this period you continue using the homeopathic spray each day while following the Cura Romana Food Plan to the letter.

The body begins to shed unwanted fat rapidly. By Day 24 you are likely to have lost between 11 and 23 pounds (5–9.5 kilos).

During the last three days (Days 22–24 inclusive) you will continue on the Food Plan, but without taking the homeopathic spray – which needs to clear from the body before you enter Consolidation.

After three weeks on the hCG+Food Plan programme your system will have become very clean and highly responsive to whatever foods you eat afterwards. This is a tremendous opportunity to learn which foods work well for your body and which do not, and for you to make powerful, positive choices so that you can maintain your new body long into the future.

Next 6 Weeks: Consolidation

This part of the Cura Romana programme lasts six weeks. **It is the most important part of your Cura Romana journey as it focuses on making your weightloss last.** You will not be taking the homeopathic spray during this six-week period.

Now is the time when the body integrates the positive shifts and balances in the body and brain instigated during the hCG+Food period. The goal of Consolidation is to make the new way your fat-control centre has learned to function a normal part of your life, leaving behind the abnormal functioning that once caused you to gain weight and hold on to it.

Consolidation stabilizes the weight you've lost, helps strengthen your body and creates greater awareness of the foods on which your body thrives, as well as those which undermine your well-being. During this period you will discover a new relationship to the foods you eat and establish new patterns for making your new body size and shape last.

Big Pay-offs

Not only does Cura Romana remove unwanted fat quickly and easily, it strengthens health and greatly alleviates or eliminates many chronic medical conditions, rejuvenating the body in medically measurable ways. More about all this anon.

Thanks to the work of A. T. W. Simeons and the recent discovery that homeopathic hCG can replace the medical version of his original Protocol, a whole new world of weightloss has come into being. The metabolic processes involved in the Roman Cure are now available to anyone. They are nothing short of revolutionary. Yet they were discovered and the Protocol created more than half a century ago. It's time to meet the man who made it all possible.

THE CREATOR

ALFRED THEODORE WILLIAM SIMEONS, MD, was among the most gifted medical researchers of the twentieth century. Born in London in 1900, he graduated *summa cum laude* in medicine from Heidelberg University. After postgraduate studies in Germany and Switzerland, he took up an appointment at a large hospital in Dresden where he began to study tropical diseases. He joined the School of Tropical Medicine in Hamburg, became fascinated by the subject, then spent two years in Africa. There he invented a method for identifying the various strains of malarial parasites in the blood which became known as Simeons' Stain. It is still used today for the same purpose. Simeons also discovered the injectable antimalarial drug atebrin, which is still used to treat the disease.

Achievements and Awards

In 1931 Simeons left Africa and went to practise and live in India. There, for sixteen years, he also held a number of government posts during the latter stages of the British Raj and after independence he was declared a consultant to the government of India.

Throughout the Second World War Simeons researched bubonic

plague and leprosy. Troubled by the conditions in which lepers had long been forced to live, he designed and built a unique model leprosy asylum. It provided pleasant surroundings, shady trees, sound accommodation and good ventilation. Far ahead of its time, it later became an All-India centre for the disease. During his years in India he began writing a novel about a leper's life; it was eventually published by Knopf under the title *The Mask of a Lion*. Simeons' contributions to medicine were so significant that he was decorated by The Queen, who presented him with the Red Cross Order of Merit for his achievements.

While in India, Simeons had developed a fascination with two other areas of medicine which were to become the focus of his medical work for the rest of his life – psychosomatic medicine and a quest for the cause and cure of obesity. In 1949 he left India with his wife and two sons, and went to live and work in Rome. There, as a consultant at the Salvator Mundi International Hospital, he continued to probe into relationships between mind and body, while intensifying his primary research and clinical work in his search for an answer to obesity. He died in Rome at the age of seventy.

The Writer

Simeons was the author of numerous articles, scientific papers and books on health and medicine. He wrote both in German and in his native English.

The Road of the Forgotten (in German, 1950).
The Mask of a Lion (a novel, 1952).
*Man's Presumptuous Brain: An Evolutionary
    Interpretation of Psychosomatic Disease* (1960).
Ramlal (a novel, 1965).
The Development of the Human Brain (in German, 1967).
Pounds and Inches: A New Approach to Obesity (privately
    published for doctors and patients, 1967).
Food, Facts and Fables: The Origins of Human Nutrition
    (1968).

Fat-boy Secrets

In India, Simeons had treated a number of 'fat boys' – youths suffering from a well-known medical condition known as Frölich's syndrome or *hypothalamic infantilism-obesity*. This condition develops as a result of malfunction or damage in the hypothalamus. It is characterized by an under-development of male genitals and the appearance of feminine sex characteristics, including an *abnormal distribution of fat* on the body. The bodies of these youths look more female than male. They have long, slender hands, breasts, large hips, bottoms and thighs, as well as striations on the skin, knock-knees and undescended testicles. Low blood pressure, low body temperature and low blood sugar are also characteristic of the condition. So are distortions in the function of the brain's appetite-control centre, which gives them ravenous appetites and leads to chronic over-eating and extreme obesity.

The accepted way of treating this condition had been to inject the boys twice a week with several hundred IUs of human chorionic gonadotrophin. This form of treatment was originally developed as a result of animal experiments showing that, when pure hCG is injected into immature rats, they become sexually precocious.

The treatment was reasonably effective. However, Simeons was faced with a problem. HCG is expensive and the number of youths suffering from Frölich's syndrome whom he needed to treat was high. He was determined to discover a more effective treatment – the best treatment possible – at a much lower cost. He began a clinical study to discover what the smallest effective dose of hCG would be.

Three significant findings emerged from his research:

1 He discovered that giving the youths a retention enema containing a mere 300cc of hCG taken from the fresh urine of a pregnant woman brought excellent results.

2 He established that small daily doses were equally as

effective as the much larger weekly doses that he and his colleagues had been using.

3 He was greatly surprised to find that these small doses, given daily, brought an end – once and for all – to the insatiable hunger and chronic over-eating which continually plagued the youths. And, although their weights did not change, the shape of their bodies altered dramatically. Abnormal fat deposits on their hips, chests and thighs – responsible for feminizing their bodies – diminished and then disappeared.

Simeons asked himself an important question: if shape-distorting, abnormal fat could be set on the move as a consequence of small doses of hCG, causing it to transit from one part of the body to another, was it possible that, under the right circumstances, these fat deposits could be encouraged to *burn up* at the same time? Could these abnormal fat deposits, as they burned, be turned into usable life energy? If so, might they – at least in part – replace the body's need to rely on energy taken in the form of calories from foods eaten?

To test out these hypotheses, he gave the youths a small daily dose of hCG and put them on a diet that restricted their food intake to 500 calories a day. To his surprise, the boys shed a pound or more a day from abnormal fat deposits *without hunger.* They were able to go about their daily activities without fatigue. Their flesh remained firm. Their skin glowed with health while the shape of their bodies normalized. Negative side-effects? There were none.

A Fat Obsession

By the time he died, Simeons had spent more than forty years of his life grappling with obesity – its causes, its manifestations and its biochemical and physiological characteristics. His clear-headedness and practical methods never failed him. He never allowed himself to get side-tracked by facile theories. He refused to buy into the belief –

still widely held – that people get fat because they eat too much or because they have no willpower.

> **Simeons says:** *When obese patients are accused of cheating, gluttony, lack of willpower, greed and sexual complexes, the strong become indignant and decide that modern medicine is a fraud, while the weak just give up the struggle in despair. In either case the result is the same: a further weight gain [and] resignation to an abominable fate.*

Simeons felt sure that obesity must develop because of a functional disorder in some area of the body. With each year that passed he grew more determined to find out where the malfunction causing people to get fat was located. He knew first hand that slimming diets were not the answer. Putting a patient on a weightloss diet was no more useful than putting a sticking plaster on a skinned knee badly in need of cleaning and disinfecting. He saw how people would lose weight temporarily then, in virtually every case, regain the fat lost later. Year by year he evaluated every new theory on obesity that appeared in the medical literature. He investigated each new method. He checked out every hopeful lead. All led to disappointing results.

> **Simeons says:** *The tendency to accumulate abnormal fat is a very definite metabolic disorder probably connected with one or more glands or organs, much as Grave's disease and Hashimoto's condition are the results of a malfunction of the thyroid gland and diabetes is the result of a badly functioning pancreas.*

If there was an abnormal gland or organ that was responsible for obesity, where was it to be found? Long before, he had developed a habit of writing down and reviewing each clinical case as though it were an odd piece in the vast jigsaw puzzle known as obesity. Gradually some of these pieces began to coalesce. He put together a workable hypothesis. Whether the hypothesis represented some ulti-mate truth mattered less to him than whether it provided an intellectually satisfying interpretation of what happens to the chronically overweight body that he would be able either to validate or to reject. It would have to stand up to the onslaught of clinical facts, as well as to provide him with a firm foundation upon which the results of obesity treatment could be accurately tested. Twenty years into his search, the complete picture of obesity began to emerge.

Thanks to the fat boys

Simeons remembered his work with the fat boys in India. He recalled the way their bodies had changed shape on the highly restricted low-calorie diet he had put them on while giving them tiny daily doses of hCG. He remembered how easy they had found it to stick to his specific very low-calorie diet and the way they had no need to struggle with hunger. These things, he concluded, could be explained only by the fact that their abnormal fat deposits were being turned into usable energy. The energy made available as fat was used up replaced the extra calories they would have needed had they been on the very low-calorie diet *without* the help of hCG. He recalled that there were no negative side-effects – only positive ones. 'Might the same treatment be useful to overweight men and women?' he asked himself.

At the hospital in Rome, he began to experiment with the method on obese men and women. It took a few hundred cases for him to be certain that the physical transformations he had seen in the fat boys were equally apparent in the treatment of the obese. His patients lost weight rapidly on two meals a day of 250 calories each. They experi-enced so little hunger that at times even the small amount of food they were supposed to be eating felt more than they could manage. Often they reported a sense of having just eaten a huge meal. Equally rewarding was the way in which the distorted body shapes of his obesity patients normalized as abnormal fat deposits diminished.

The body transformed

Simeons was sure he had discovered something important. But he continued to work quietly and steadily, always refining his treatment in an attempt to make it virtually foolproof. One day he realized that, probably for the first time in medical history, he had devised a way of providing his patients with a pathway to *permanent* weightloss. Cura Romana – the name that would be given to his discovery by patients and doctors throughout the world – had finally been born.

Not until January 1954 did Simeons tell the medical world a little about his discoveries. As soon as he made his method of obesity treatment available to the medical community, it triggered a tsunami of controversy which, even now – more than half a century on – continues to rage.

THE SKINNY ON FAT

VALID DISCOVERIES IN medicine depend on the ability of researchers to make accurate observations in relation to the subject they are studying. As famous French science historian Claude Bernard pointed out more than 150 years ago, 'To have an idea about a natural phenomenon, we must first of all *observe* it. All human knowledge is limited to working back from observed effects to their cause.' Scientists with preconceived notions assume that they already know the cause and this makes it impossible for them to make valid observations. They are only able to see what they *expect* to see.

This is what has been happening with virtually all the obesity research carried out in the past seventy years. Researchers have been taking as a *given* a false assumption that, by now, has all the earmarks of fundamentalist dogma. This mistaken doctrine continues to blind them to the truth. To express it in the words of the Surgeon General of the United States, 'overweight and obesity are the result of excess calorie consumption and/or inadequate physical activity'.

This notion has reigned supreme amongst doctors, research scientists and the media until this day. If you take as much time to plough through scientific papers as I have, you can't help but conclude that this doctrine is completely false. As the prestigious National Academy of Sciences report *Diet and Health* points out, 'most studies comparing normal and overweight people suggest that those who are overweight eat fewer calories than those of normal weight'. Yet this dangerous false assumption continues to rule them and us.

Had Claude Bernard lived half a century later, he would have celebrated A. T. W. Simeons' methods of investigation. Simeons was a master of observation and practicality. He refused to be side-tracked by such facile beliefs about obesity.

> **Simeons says:** *What I have to say is, in essence, the views distilled out of forty years of grappling with the fundamental problems of obesity, its causes, its symptoms, and its very nature. In these many years of specialized work, thousands of cases have passed through my hands and were carefully studied. Every new theory, every new method, every promising lead was considered, experimentally screened and critically evaluated as soon as it became known. I felt that we were merely nibbling at the fringe of a great problem.*

Simeons postulated that a tendency to accumulate excess fat was likely to be the *result* of some metabolic disorder – not its *cause*. If obesity in its many forms were indeed due to an abnormal functioning of some part of the body, then each and every ounce of abnormally accumulated fat would have to have been the result of this functional abnormality. He set out to find what it was.

> **Simeons says:** *Persons suffering from this particular disorder will get fat regardless of whether they eat excessively, normally or less than normal. A person who is free of the disorder will never get fat, even if he frequently overeats.*

To identify the cause and effective treatment for obesity he faced four major challenges:

1 He had to study the origins of obesity from an evolutionary point of view; to discover when in human history it had begun and, if possible, to determine what changes in man's way of living could have brought it about.

2 He needed to investigate the various kinds of fat in the human body – both normal and abnormal – and to learn as much as possible about each in relation to weight gain and weightloss.

3 If, as he suspected, obesity was a functional disorder, he would need to identify in what organ, gland or area of the body this metabolic distortion had taken place.

4 Finally, it would be necessary to determine a way of restoring normal function to this locus, thereby allowing the body to shed its excess fat and preventing future regains.

How We Got Fat

Simeons observed that obesity occurs only in human beings and a few domestic animals – the latter as a result of selective breeding and unnatural feeding. In wild animals – even in animals that build up stores of fat in autumn to prepare for winter hibernation – the abnormal characteristics seen in human obesity never appear. He noticed that potentially or overtly obese parents can, and often do, pass on a tendency to gain fat to their children. This does not necessarily condemn someone with this genetic inheritance to accumulating abnormal fat. However, when this trait is inherited from both parents, a young child will frequently begin to accumulate abnormal fat at an early age. If the tendency is transferred by a single parent, more often it reveals itself only later in life – if at all.

Genetic inheritance

Wild animals eat only when they are hungry. They never eat more than their bodies need for the moment. Recent archaeological and anthropological research indicates that Paleolithic man – whose genes we have inherited – lived the same way. Our ancestors were hunter-gatherers going back a million years or more. They ate when food was available and fasted when it was not. As a result, they ate a little and never continually. It's important to listen to our bodies; to eat when we are hungry and to refrain from eating when we are not.

> **Simeons says:** *In the early Neolithic times another change took place which may well account for the fact that today nearly all inherited dispositions sooner or later develop into manifest obesity. This change was the institution of regular meals. In pre-Neolithic times, man ate only when he was hungry and only as much as he required to still the pangs of hunger. Moreover, much of his food was raw and all of it was unrefined. He roasted his meat, but he did not boil it, as he had no pots, and what little he may have grubbed from the Earth and picked from the trees, he ate as he went along.*

Countless studies in paleopathology have shown that our primitive ancestors lived on a diet of flesh foods and fats together with whatever fibre-rich vegetables, herbs, seeds, roots and berries were available. It is estimated that between 60 and 90 per cent of the calories early men and women took in came in the form of large and small game animals, eggs, birds, reptiles and insects. Starchy vegetables (such as the modern potato), grains and modern-day rice did not exist.

Examination of the remains of these hunter-gatherers shows that early man had superb bone structure, flawless teeth and heavy musculature. It was during the hunter-gatherer period that our own biological terrain was formed. And, whether our political and religious leanings like it or not, this protein-orientated, flesh-based fare is the diet on which our bodies appear to thrive. Why? It is on such a diet that the forces of natural selection have refined and moulded us to function best. Our physiology has been determined by genetic programming which cares nothing about the individual. It is concerned only with our survival as a species. To put it another way, we have been genetically programmed to eat like this for thousands of centuries.

It takes between 40,000 and 100,000 years to bring about a single significant genetic change. Our system still functions very much as did those of our Paleolithic ancestors. As a result, we are designed to thrive when we eat relatively small quantities of food and frequently fast for 12 hours or more.

When Neolithic man appeared on the scene between 10,700 and 9,400 BCE, bringing with him the agricultural revolution and seeding the development of cities and the growth of what we call civilization, massive changes started to take place in man's life and diet. They were marked by a high degree of urbanization. Collect people together en masse and you need to feed them from a relatively small area. Farming and animal husbandry became widespread. This meant relying heavily on carbohydrate foods in the form of starchy vegetables and cereal crops, like rice and wheat. Gradually, cereals, fruits and starchy vegetables came to play a large part in human nutrition. Man's protein intake decreased dramatically.

Obesity begins

Not only did agricultural man add grains, legumes and milk to his diet, the growth of farming meant he began to live a more sedentary life than had his hunter-gatherer ancestors. This too was great for the development of civilization – but not without a cost to his body and his health. By the time the agricultural revolution was in full swing – about 4,000 years ago – degeneration had begun in the human body. Men and women shrank in height. Dental decay and malformation of the jaw appeared. Disease epidemics began to shorten natural human lifespan. This time in history marks the beginning of what we nowadays call the 'diseases of civilization' – and, most important of all, the beginning of obesity.

> **Simeons says:** *The whole structure of man's omnivorous digestive tract is, like that of an ape, rat or pig, adjusted to the continual nibbling of tidbits. It is not suited to occasional gorging as is, for instance, the intestine of the carnivorous cat family. Thus the institution of regular meals, particularly of food digested and assimilated rapidly, placed a great burden on modern man's ability to cope with large quantities of food suddenly pouring into his system from the intestinal tract.*

The institution of regular meals meant that man was obliged to eat more than his body required at the moment of eating in order to tide him over until the next meal. Cereal- and grain-based foods, which were quick and easy to digest, began to flood the body with nourishment he could not make use of at the time of eating. Somehow, somewhere, this surplus had to be stored. As time passed, some of the human race developed a tendency to store this excess food in the form of fat. Since the dietary changes had taken place so rapidly from an evolutionary point of view, their bodies could not handle them. As centuries passed, we ate more and more of these rapidly assimilated foods. In Venice in the fifteenth century sugar was refined for the first time. Since then, things have only become worse. Ninety per cent of the packaged convenience foods we eat are manufactured using these fast-uptake foods. Meanwhile we grow fatter and fatter. Our modern habits of eating masses of cooked food replete with sugar, cereals and starchy vegetables make our bodies assimilate foods so fast that we cannot effectively turn them into usable energy.

The Good, the Bad and the Ugly

Your body's ability to lay down fat is a perfectly normal and necessary strategy for survival. After all, fat has the highest caloric value of any food type. It is the perfect way for our bodies to store food reserves in the smallest possible space. When we eat plenty of food, the body stores away any surplus it does not need at the time. If all works well metabolically, this stored fat is meant to be kept on hand, ready to supply sustenance whenever the body is in need of more food than happens to be available. If it doesn't work well, we get fat.

After years of studying obesity, Simeons identified three kinds of fat in the human body. Two of them are normal and *essential*. The third is both *inessential* and abnormal. Only the inessential, abnormal fat creates obesity.

You can easily identify the difference when you look under a microscope. The first kind of normal fat – also known as *visceral* or *structural* fat – acts like upholstery or packing-material to cushion our internal organs. It guards delicate structures such as the bladder, the spleen, the kidneys and the eyeballs by embedding them in soft elastic tissue. It also protects the coronary arteries, helps keep the skin firm and smooth and creates the vital cushion of firm fat under the heels of the feet without which we would be unable to walk without pain.

The second variety of normal fat is evenly distributed throughout the body. It provides an equally important reserve of energy so that, when there is a lack of food or a famine, we are able to call on this reserve to fuel our metabolism and keep us going. Both these fats – structural and reserve – are important to the well-being of any man or woman. And even if your body chooses to store these essential fats to capacity, they will never make you obese. A healthy, well-fed body can function perfectly well for a limited time subsisting only on its normal fat reserves.

The third kind of fat is inessential and *abnormal* fat you see in the build-up of the adipose deposits which distort our bodies. It creates beer bellies on men and spreading waistlines, thighs and bottoms on women. It is these inessential fat deposits that result in obesity. Theoretically, one would expect this kind of fat to function as a 'reserve of fuel' just as normal fat does. The problem is that in people with a tendency to gain weight, this non-essential fat gets 'locked away' beyond reach so that, even when your body needs energy, you are unable to access it.

When we go on slimming diets, or on fasts, instead of being able to tap into this kind of inessential fat, we often shed our normal reserves as well. This is one reason yo-yo dieters suffer such frustration. What's worse, if we stay on one of these diets, it can result in a loss of essential, structural fat, undermining our health.

> **Simeons says:** *When an obese patient tries to reduce by starving himself, he will first lose his normal fat reserves. When these are exhausted he begins to burn up structural fat, and only as a last resort will the body yield its abnormal reserves, though by that time the patient usually feels so weak and hungry that the diet is abandoned. It is just for this reason that obese patients complain that when they diet they lose the wrong fat. They feel famished and tired and their face becomes drawn and haggard, but their belly, hips, thighs and upper arms show little improvement. The fat they have come to detest stays on and the fat they need to cover their bones gets less and less. Their skin wrinkles and they look old and miserable. And that is one of the most frustrating and depressing experiences a human being can have.*

When it comes to a chronically overweight or obese body, the normal mechanisms of fat-storage and fat-burning have become grossly distorted. Simeons liked to describe this phenomenon using a simile which likens body fat to money. Our essential fat supply – the structural and reserve fats – are like our possessions: homes, cars, gold, money, belongings. The inessential fat that the body stores *should* behave as excess income. It would be great if it did – if we were able to draw on it for energy whenever we needed it. But in the case of someone overweight or who gains weight easily, a distortion in the body's fat-management system prevents their being able to turn this fat into energy. Instead, it gets locked away in what Simeons refers to as a 'deposit account', rendering the potential energy it holds unavailable. The implications of this are vast. For an overweight man or woman it creates a situation in which, although he or she feels hungry, much of what is eaten in an attempt to quell that hunger gets turned into fat and stashed away beyond reach. Therefore eating food often doesn't assuage their hunger. Nor does it provide the energy they long for. As a result, they can remain low in vitality yet still crave more food. This produces a vicious cycle: hunger leads to more eating, the storing of more fat and the perpetuation of cravings which are never satisfied.

> **Simeons says:** *Obese patients only feel physically well as long as they are stationary or gaining weight. They may feel guilty, owing to the lethargy and indolence always associated with obesity. They may feel ashamed of what they have been led to believe is a lack of control. They may feel horrified by the appearance of their nude body and the tightness of their clothes. But they have a primitive feeling of animal content which turns to misery and suffering as soon as they make a resolute attempt to reduce. For this there are sound reasons.*

All Change

To recap: the most significant change to human diets in two million years began with the agricultural revolution, when man went from a carbohydrate-poor to a carbohydrate-rich diet, as cereals and quickly digestible starches entered our diet. The more that these carbohydrates have become refined in the past 300 years, the more problems they have caused us, not only in terms of burgeoning obesity worldwide, but also in the development of the chronic degenerative diseases of civilization.

More recently, the overwhelming increase in sugars and fructose – especially in the form of corn syrup – in so many convenience foods has become a major contributor on both counts. In the eighteenth century we ate between 10 and 20 pounds of sugar per person per year. Today we consume between 150 and 212 pounds per capita. Yet the vast majority of obesity researchers continue to insist that fat accumulation is a mere question of a 'calories in, calories out' situation, demanding little more than willpower and regular exercise to sort out. Meanwhile, according to World Health Organization statistics, more than a billion adults throughout the world are now overweight. Obesity rates have 'risen threefold or more since 1980 in some areas of North America, the United Kingdom, Eastern Europe, the Middle East, the Pacific Islands, Australasia, and China.'

An important observation attributed to the German philosopher Arthur Schopenhauer is highly appropriate to the thousands of research projects which remain unsuccessful in establishing the cause of and cure for obesity as a result of the unfounded 'calories in, calories out' assumption on which they continue to be based: 'All truth passes through three stages. First, it is ridiculed. Second, it is violently opposed. Third, it is accepted as being self-evident.'

It is time for mainstream science to move beyond the first and second stages that Schopenhauer describes if it is to bring to an end the expanding obesity epidemic plaguing the world, as well as the chronic illness and deep suffering it engenders. Meanwhile, let's look at the third and fourth challenges facing Simeons in his search for the cause of and cure for obesity: identifying where in the body the functional disorder for which he had been searching was located; and finding a way of restoring a healthy balance that would enable the body to shed its inessential fat stores and keep them off.

THE REVELATIONS

I N HIS LONGING to determine which organ, gland or system is responsible for body-fat control, Simeons investigated every theory one by one. He worked out that obesity is not the result of a faulty mechanism in the sex glands, the adrenals, the pituitary or the thyroid. What he found in relation to the thyroid in the process is valuable in its own right. Until this day doctors have gone on prescribing thyroid medication to overweight people on the assumption that, if a person is hypothyroid, it is necessary to give thyroid hormones to solve their weight problem. Unfortunately it doesn't solve the problem. Yet the practice lives on.

> **Simeons says:** *When it was discovered that the thyroid gland controls the rate at which body-fuel is consumed, it was thought that by administering thyroid gland to obese patients their abnormal fat deposits could be burned up more rapidly. This too proved to be entirely disappointing, because as we now know, these abnormal deposits take no part in the body's energy-turnover – they are inaccessibly locked away. Thyroid medication merely forces the body to*

consume its normal fat reserves, which are already depleted in obese patients, and then to break down structurally essential fat without touching the abnormal deposits. In this way a patient may be brought to the brink of starvation in spite of having a hundred pounds of fat to spare. Thus any weightloss brought about by thyroid medication is always at the expense of fat of which the body is in dire need.

Fat-bank Controlling

It was largely thanks to his years of work treating youths with Frölich's syndrome in India that Simeons was able to pinpoint that the body's fat-control and fat-bank regulating system is located in an area of the brain known as the *diencephalon*. A complex of structures including the thalamus, hypothalamus and pituitary, the diencephalon is probably the most sensitive and complex locus of control in the whole body. It governs the central nervous system, our hormones, emotions, stress and mood. It oversees our autonomic nervous system, heart rate, the urinary system, blood pressure, body temperature, fluid and electrolyte balance, sexuality and sleep cycles. Within the complex that forms the diencephalon, the hypothalamus is the most important gland when it comes to our experience of hunger and thirst. With the help of the other members of the diencephalon team, and the neural and hormonal connections they make with the rest of the body, the hypothalamus decides whether your body lays down more inessential fat as well as how and when it lets go of it.

As far back as seventy years ago there was much experimental evidence to confirm Simeons' findings. Since then, more has come to light to support them. When, for instance, the diencephalon in the brain of a healthy animal is mechanically destroyed by a needle inserted through its skull, the animal invariably develops a gigantic appetite. It also starts to accumulate abnormal fat at a rate of knots – creating a condition virtually identical to that of human obesity.

Again, Simeons often compared the way the diencephalon deals with these issues with banking. It manages our fat deposits and with-drawals the way a bank manages our money. When you take in more caloric energy from your food than your body needs at any moment, the surplus gets deposited in your 'current account'. This current account holds *normal* fat deposits, from which your body can *withdraw* caloric energy when it needs to. But when, for any reason (such as those listed below), fat deposits become more frequent than your withdrawals, a point is reached which goes beyond the diencephalon's banking capacity to hold them in such a way that they continue to be accessible to you.

> **Simeons says:** *Just as a banker might suggest to a wealthy client that instead of accumulating a large and unmanageable current account he should invest his surplus capital, the body appears to establish a fixed deposit into which all surplus funds go but from which they can no longer be withdrawn by the procedure used in a current account. In this way the diencephalic 'fat-bank' frees itself from all work which goes beyond its normal banking capacity. The onset of obesity dates from the moment the diencephalon adopts this labour-saving ruse. Once a fixed deposit has been established the normal fat reserves are held at a minimum, while every available surplus is locked away in the fixed deposit and is therefore taken out of normal circulation.*

In people who have *not* inherited a tendency to obesity, as soon as the limit of their diencephalic fat-banking capacity is reached, the hypothalamus automatically curbs their appetite. They do not gain further weight. In those of us genetically predisposed to weight gain, this mechanism does not shut off appetite and limit further weight gain. In effect, it does not function in the way it was meant to do.

There appear to be three major factors lying behind fat-banking errors through which obesity can become manifest.

1 Genetic inheritance Someone's diencephalic fat-banking capacity may have been abnormally low from the time they were born. A tendency to obesity can run in families, manifesting in some of the children but not in others. Two sisters, born of the same parents and eating the same food at the same table, can grow up with one of them becoming fat while the other stays lean.

2 Functional disorders of the diencephalon Simeons observed that a lowering of someone's previously normal fat-banking capacity can occur when the body has been making excessive demands on one or more of the members of the diencephalon – say the thalamus. This gland then attempts to increase its functional capacity at the expense of the other members, upsetting their balance as well and leading to weight gain. Menopause, a traumatic event or even prolonged stress can trigger this.

3 Sudden excess exhausts fat bank During the Second World War, 6,000 emaciated Polish refugees were moved to camps in India, then fed normal British rations. As a result, 85 per cent of them became obese within three months.

Simeons says: *In a person eating coarse and unrefined food, the digestion is slow and only a little nourishment at a time is assimilated from the intestinal tract. When such a person is suddenly able to obtain highly refined foods such as sugar, white flour, butter and oil these are so rapidly digested and assimilated that the rush of incoming fuel which occurs at every meal may eventually overpower the diencephalic regulatory mechanisms and thus lead to obesity. This is commonly seen in the poor man who*

suddenly becomes rich enough to buy the more expensive
refined foods, though his total caloric intake remains the
same or is even less than before.

Given that in the past fifty years obesity has become a worldwide epidemic as a result of our massive consumption of convenience foods, fast foods and meals based on highly refined foods, it is likely that this exhaustion of the fat-banking system has been occurring in the bodies of literally millions of unsuspecting people, thereby engendering widespread degenerative conditions. The saddest part of all this is that they often have no idea why this is happening to them.

Thanks to Simeons' clinical experiments in applying variations of his 'fat-boy treatment' to overweight men and women over many years, he was able to formulate a workable method for restoring good function to the diencephalon's fat-banking in his overweight patients, thereby enabling their bodies to shed their abnormal, inessential fat reserves swiftly and with little or no hunger. He did this by combining two carefully honed sources of power – hCG and his highly specific Food Plan.

Enter the Hero

HCG is an acronym for *human chorionic gonadotrophin* – a protein-based hormone often called the *pregnancy hormone*. It starts being made in a woman's body seven or eight days after conception. This is the hormone that we rely on when we buy a common pregnancy test from a pharmacy. The line which turns blue when you dip the strip into your urine indicates that a woman is pregnant because the strip reacts to the presence of hCG in her urine.

In 1928, hCG was discovered in the urine of pregnant women by German scientists Selmar Aschheim and Bernhard Zondek. In naming their discovery, they used the words 'chorionic' because it was produced by the chorium of the placenta and 'gonadotrophin' to indicate that hCG acts on the gonads – that is, the ovaries and testes. They came up with the name because giving the substance to laboratory animals provoked ovulation in the females, but it was an unfortunate misnomer. It has led the world to believe that hCG is some kind of sex hormone – a steroid related to oestrogen or testosterone, for example. This is untrue.

Unique Hormone

The word 'hormone' was coined in 1921 and comes from the Greek meaning 'to act through distance'. It is used to describe substances secreted by an organ or gland, then carried to a distant part of the body to act. The hormone insulin, for instance, is made in the pancreas then sent all over the body to do its work. HCG is very different from the fat-based steroids and sex hormones – the oestrogens, progesterone, testosterone and other steroid hormones, such as cortisone, made in the adrenals. HCG is a *protein-based* hormone which, like insulin, human growth hormone and leptin, plays important roles in regulating energy intake and expenditure, appetite and metabolism. Actually, hCG is the largest and most complex glycoprotein present in the human body. It holds some 300 amino acids in its molecular structure.

New life brought to birth

In pregnancy, hCG helps keep the *corpus luteum* strong and healthy. This is the part of an ovary central to the production of the high levels of progesterone needed to prevent miscarriage and to keep the developing baby safe until it is ready to be born. HCG also provides a woman's body with heightened immunity while she is holding new life within her womb.

During pregnancy, the levels of hCG in her body increase week by week until, by the time she is three months pregnant, she is likely to have as many as 300,000 IU of this remarkable hormone in every millilitre of her circulating blood supply. If she is carrying twins, the levels will be even higher. The presence of this protein-based hormone in the body strongly affects the diencephalon's fat-banking.

> **Simeons says:** *Pregnancy seems to be the only normal human condition in which the diencephalic fat banking capacity is unlimited. It is only during pregnancy that fixed fat deposits can be transferred back into the normal current account and freely drawn upon to make up for any nutritional deficit. During pregnancy, every ounce of reserve fat is placed at the disposal of the growing foetus . . . There is considerable evidence to suggest that it is the hCG produced in large quantities in the placenta which brings about this diencephalic change.*

All good news

Not only does hCG exert no *negative* side-effects on a pregnant woman's body, but it brings a number of medically *positive* side-effects. These are in addition to its role in helping prevent miscarriage. These health-enhancing effects are also experienced by men and women on Cura Romana.

- it helps regulate metabolism
- it brings greater emotional stability
- it improves sleep patterns
- it boosts mental clarity
- it enhances energy
- it brings relief from aches and pains

Probably the most important function hCG performs in a pregnant woman's body is an evolutionary one: it directs her body to draw upon her own fat stores as a means of feeding the placenta and foetus.

What is interesting – and probably not yet known in Simeons' time – is that hCG appears to be a ubiquitous, natural substance which takes part in life processes on a large scale. It is not only produced in the body of a pregnant woman, it is also found in small amounts within almost all normal human tissues – male or female, pregnant or not. Even plants and bacteria synthesize hCG. Having worked with it on Cura Romana and witnessed the enhancements it can bring to people in its homeopathic form, I have a strong sense that it may, in some as yet unexplained capacity, also act as some kind of communicator between spirit and body. More about this possibility in 'The Transformation' section of the book (see page 308).

When it comes to simple weightloss, Simeons' most important discovery was that, in the bodies of overweight men and women, small quantities of hCG were able to perform a feat similar to what it brings about in a pregnant woman's body. It enables overweight bodies to access caloric energy from inessential adipose tissues and burn it up, producing life-energy for use.

A mere 250 IU of hCG coupled with his carefully designed 500-calorie diet reduces body weight rapidly, safely and with little or no hunger. The quantity needed to accomplish this is incredibly small when you consider that a woman excretes up to 1,000,000 IU of hCG a day in her urine. Despite the limited number of calories his patients were taking in, they reported little or no hunger. People were able to carry on living normal, vital lives. The only thing that was required of them on the Cura Romana programme was that they follow the dietary Protocol with precision.

What You Need to Know

Simeons drew three important conclusions out of his clinical experience with more than 6,000 patients on Cura Romana:

● Men and women given hCG lose the same amount of weight as those who follow the same very low-calorie diet without the help of hCG. However, the weightloss from those on hCG plus the food Protocol is drawn from *inessential* fat deposits. By contrast, weight lost on the diet but *without* the support of hCG results in a significant loss of lean body mass and *essential, structural* fat, both of which the body requires for health.

● People treated with hCG remain vital and in good spirits throughout the programme.

● The foods that make up the very low-calorie diet are of great importance to the success of the programme. The slightest deviation from this exacting Protocol can bring unfavourable results. Thanks to the way hCG+Food Plan mobilizes fat mass, body contours change rapidly, restoring the body to its more normal shape and size.

Instead of getting saggy and loose as it does on conventional diets, their skin grew firmer. Sleep improved. So did premenstrual troubles and menopausal symptoms. The way Cura Romana accomplishes all this is, of course, highly complex and still little understood. But Simeons is clear that, fundamentally, it acts upon the hypothalamus and other members of the diencephalon, metabolizing inessential fat stores and restoring greater neurological and hormonal balance.

Medical research has chosen to ignore his explanation. Since Aschheim and Zondek isolated hCG in 1923, thousands of scientific articles have appeared in medical journals concerning human chorionic gonadotrophin. Most talk about using massive doses of hCG as a treatment for infertility or Frölich's syndrome. However, little research has been carried out to confirm the effectiveness of hCG as a treatment in other conditions. Meanwhile, it continues to be used by forward-thinking physicians in the successful treatment of a wide variety of illnesses. These include asthma, gastritis, neurosis, heart damage, hyperlipidaemia (the presence of excess fats in the blood), hypercholesterolaemia (higher than normal levels of cholesterol in the blood), eczema, glaucoma, alcoholism, psychoses, osteopenia (mild thinning of bone mass, but not as severe as osteoporosis), cancer, thalassaemia (a genetically based blood condition) and rheumatic conditions.

HCG has been used to slow down and arrest the spread of cancer-like tumours appearing in AIDS patients – known as Kaposi's sarcoma. With so few articles written to explore the vast therapeutic potential that this natural, non-toxic, protein-based hormone appears to offer – including the treatment of obesity – a great potential for health improvement is being ignored. Not long ago, the International Society for Alternative Uses of hCG (ISAUC) was established in Buenos Aires with the intention of encouraging greater scientific investigation into the largely untapped therapeutic potential hCG offers. One hopes that it will not turn out to be the only voice crying in the wilderness for more work to be done exploring this important substance.

A future for hCG

Meanwhile, some of the reports and unproved assumptions that have arisen from animal studies and from the clinical experience of doctors who have worked with patients on Cura Romana point to findings too important to be ignored. Here are a few:

- Obesity is still a poorly understood disease which originates in the hypothalamic region of the diencephalon. It is the result of damage to this area, an imbalance of neuropeptide concentration in this region or some other distorting influence.
- As a result of this disorder and the widespread imbalances it engenders, the body accumulates inessential fat with little restraint.
- In obese people, the deposits of inessential fat which distort body shape behave quite differently to normal fat deposits.

They are also highly resistant to conventional weightloss diets.

- Animal studies show that, when given small doses of hCG, this protein-based hormone accumulates in the hypothalamic region of the brain.
- HCG intensifies the metabolism of brown fat – the kind of adipose tissue which, when activated, helps to burn fat in the body.
- Thanks to its hypothalamic action, hCG also slows down the formation of new fat cells in the body.

Brown Fat

Three new studies that have appeared recently in *The New England Journal of Medicine* show that brown fat in humans has the potential to fight obesity. 'It is, in a sense, the discovery of a new organ,' said Sven Enerbäck, a researcher at the University of Gothenburg in Sweden and lead author of one of the studies.

'This is a tissue whose sole physiological purpose is to expend energy,' said Francesco S. Celi, a metabolism researcher at the National Institutes of Health, whose commentary accompanies the studies. 'That makes it an ideal target [for drugs or other measures designed to make it more active]'.

Currently, the only way to stimulate the production of brown fat is to stay cold – near shivering – for extended periods of time, reproducing the conditions that led to its evolution.

While researchers are looking at more comfortable ways to activate brown fat, don't turn down your thermostats expecting quick results just yet. According to the studies, brown fat 'might' be able to burn off 10 pounds of fat in a year when *fully stimulated*.

Simeons says: *... obesity in all its many forms is due to an abnormal functioning ... every ounce of abnormally accumulated fat is always the result of the same disorder ... Persons suffering from this particular disorder will get fat regardless of whether they eat excessively, normally or less than normal. A person who is free of the disorder will never get fat, even if he frequently overeats. Those in whom the disorder is severe will accumulate fat very rapidly, those in whom it is moderate will gradually increase in weight and those in whom it is mild may be able to keep their excess weight stationary for long periods. In all these cases a loss of weight brought about by dieting, treatments with thyroid, appetite-reducing drugs, laxatives, violent exercise, massage, or baths is only temporary and will be rapidly regained as soon as the reducing regimen is relaxed. The reason is simply that none of these measures corrects the basic disorder.*

Curiouser and Curiouser

As I mentioned earlier, the Roman Cure is not only about losing pounds. It is also about inches. Participants find that the rate at which the circumference of body parts diminishes is often more rapid than the rate at which weight is lost, especially on areas of the body resistant to fat-shedding: waists, bellies, thighs, upper arms, hips and bottoms. I suspect this is why Simeons chose to call his privately published book *Pounds and Inches*. The reason that inches diminish differently and more rapidly on Cura Romana than on conventional diets is quite simply because the programme targets inessential fat that distorts body shape.

This progressive shedding of inches and pounds always reminds me of the process by which Michelangelo described his marble-carving. 'I never sculpt anything,' he insisted. 'I chisel away the inessential marble revealing the form hidden in it all the while.' When it comes to a living body, the Roman Cure is a powerful and effective 'chisel' for clearing away inessential fat, helping to reveal the body's natural size and shape.

Beyond all this, what I continue to find most remarkable as I work with participants on Leslie Kenton's Cura Romana® is this: the parallels between Michelangelo's sculpture and the physical restructuring of the body don't appear to end with physical transformation alone. People report that, as their programme continues clearing their shape-distorting fat deposits, a similar process seems to take place in their minds. Long-held limiting beliefs, as well as the mental and emotional *static* that prevents us from making full use of our creative potentials, can also lift away. As this takes place, they report being able to tap into experiences of bliss and spiritual fulfilment not experienced before. More about this in 'The Transformation' (see page 308).

For the moment, to complete our investigations into the technical aspects of the Roman Cure, we need to take a short look at the dramas that Simeons' revelations triggered almost sixty years ago when he first announced his discoveries to the medical world. Respites in the controversy it created have been few and far between in the intervening years. If anything, the furore rages even more vehemently now than it ever has.

THE DRAMA

When A. T. W. Simeons published his brief synopsis of the Cura Romana programme in the British medical journal the *Lancet* (Vol. 2, pp. 946–47, 1954), the paper attracted the attention of doctors from around the world, many of whom journeyed to Rome to learn about it, then took what they had learned back to their own countries and began to practise it. Despite the limited number of calories their patients were taking in, they too experienced no hunger. They could carry on living their normal lives. (We will be hearing later from people who have experienced not only weightloss but the Protocol's other health benefits.)

Cura Romana's popularity was an irresistible invitation to doctors and the general public to offer their opinions on whether or not it worked and, if it did, how. Reports of phenomenal successes came flooding in, as well as aggressive attacks from those who were determined to prove it a fraud. This, in turn, led to massive confusion about the Protocol and distortions in how it was used, as well as widespread misinformation and disinformation in regard to what it was and how it worked.

In 1962 the *Journal of the American Medical Association* issued a

warning that 'continued adherence to such a drastic regimen is potentially more hazardous to the patient's health than continued obesity'.
In 1974 the FDA demanded that all companies producing hCG label
their packaging to say that it was not to be used for 'weightloss or fat
distribution'. All labelling and advertising of hCG was required to
carry a warning:

> HCG has not been demonstrated to be effective adjunctive
> therapy in the treatment of obesity. There is no substantial
> evidence that it increases weightloss beyond that resulting
> from caloric restriction [neither Simeons nor his colleagues
> ever claimed it did], that it causes a more normal distribution
> of fat, or that it decreases the hunger and discomfort associ-
> ated with calorie-restrictive diets.

Canada's Task Force on the Treatment of Obesity followed suit with its
own warning, declaring that the use of hCG for weightloss 'touches on
possible malpractice'. By this time, negative studies and government
action as good as wiped out the use of hCG for weight control in North
America. Meanwhile, in Europe, South America and elsewhere,
doctors, plastic surgeons and endocrinologists went right on using
Cura Romana and getting fine results.

The US government's Pub Med database reports more than 18,000
published papers on hCG. The majority of these articles are about hCG
– usually given in huge doses – as a fertility treatment, about its role
in pregnancy and about using it to detect malignant tumours. Almost
none examines its potential in the treatment of other illnesses – from
Kaposi's sarcoma to depression. As far as studies on hCG used for
weightloss are concerned, only a few dozen have ever been done. Most
of these were poorly designed and carried out on too small a sampling
of subjects to be statistically significant. Many seem to have been done
with a deliberate intent to prove that it does not work. Others didn't
even attempt to follow Simeons' Protocol accurately.

Bad Science

One negative study published in the *American Journal of Clinical Nutrition* during the period when Cura Romana's popularity was at its peak (Vol. 12, pp. 230–34, 1963) involved only nineteen people – ten in the treatment group and nine in the control group. For reasons difficult to fathom, researchers chose to add baked potatoes to the diet – a food absolutely forbidden on the Cura Romana Protocol. This particular study reported an average loss of 6.5 pounds in the hCG-treated group compared with an average loss of 8.8 pounds in the control group. Researchers went on to conclude that hCG does *not* cause weightloss.

Another study, published ten years later, was carried out 'to examine the effect of hCG protocol on weightloss, hunger, and a feeling of wellbeing'. It was reported in the *American Journal of Clinical Nutrition* (Vol. 26, pp. 211–18, 1973) and involved twice the number of participants. Researchers compared the hCG group with the control group and concluded that hCG *does* cause weightloss – an average of 19.96 pounds in the hCG group and only 11.05 pounds in the control group who received no hCG. Both groups showed up for a daily injection, but those in the control group were given a placebo. Neither group knew what injection they were receiving. Researchers W. L. Asher, MD, and Harold W. Harper, MD, reported that: 'The hCG group lost significantly more mean weight . . . and . . . a significantly greater mean percentage of their starting weight. The percentage of affirmative daily patient responses indicating "little or no hunger" and "feeling good to excellent" was significantly greater in the hCG group than the placebo group.'

In 1995, in a meta-analysis published in the *British Journal of Clinical Pharmacology* (Vol. 40, pp. 237–43, 1995) on the effectiveness of hCG in the treatment of obesity, researchers at Vrije University in Holland evaluated sixteen studies on the use of hCG for weightloss and reported that most had been of 'poor methodological quality'. In ordinary language, this translates as 'bad science'. Meta-analysis is an attempt to synthesize and describe results from a number of similar studies. They tend to be suspect, as the conclusions they draw depend on which studies they arbitrarily choose to include.

American research scientist Dr Dennis Clark comments that 'most research is so flawed that it is almost useless for saying anything at all with certainty'. He goes on to add, 'What I conclude regarding hCG and weightloss is based on what I have seen for myself. This includes many, many people who have had the same results that Simeons documented based on his clinical experience with thousands of patients. I have also had the same experience for myself.' Clark shed 20 pounds on the Protocol while experiencing a body-fat loss of 6 per cent in under thirty days (such a reduction in body fat is, of course, charac-teristic of Cura Romana). 'Medical researchers are apparently going to argue the merits of hCG and weightloss until the end of time, citing whatever research results support their arguments,' Clark continues. 'As a scientist myself, I have no doubt whatsoever that Simeons was right and that my body changes occurred because of hCG.'

New Kid on the Block

In 1994, long after Simeons' death, *leptin* was discovered. Leptin is also a protein hormone involved in fat-accumulation and fat-burning. And, like hCG, it communicates with the hypothalamus. Its appearance on the scene triggered yet another frenzy in the Big Pharma community. Drug companies began frantic searches for a means of turning leptin into a drug analogue which they could sell as the latest breakthrough for weightloss.

All attempts failed. Why? Because leptin has a lot in common with insulin. An overweight body is already producing masses of leptin. This creates *leptin resistance* in the cells of the hypothalamus and elsewhere, very much in the way that a high-carb/high-sugar diet creates insulin resistance resulting in *metabolic syndrome* or *Syndrome X*. Putting more leptin into an overweight body only increases a person's hunger and food cravings, inducing yet more weight gain. In the end, this discovery of leptin – considered by many to be the most important finding in regard to fat metabolism in the twentieth century – has left doctors and drug companies still at a loss as to what to do with it.

A recent discovery in regard to leptin may have relevance to our understanding of the way Cura Romana works its wonders. In the August 2007 issue of the *Journal of Endocrinology*, a paper appeared which states: 'hCG significantly stimulates the secretion of the pro-adipogenic factor, leptin, from human adipose tissue.' Nobody is able to figure out exactly the way these two protein hormones interact. However, it looks likely that leptin and hCG – together with insulin – work to determine the way the body both stores and burns fat. Animal studies have shown clearly not only that leptin and hCG influence each other, but that the effect that leptin exerts on insulin also creates an indirect response between insulin and hCG.

The important thing for you to remember is what these three protein-based hormones have in common. Excessive amounts of leptin and insulin lead to resistance, so your body cannot make good use of either. Instead of your receiving benefits from them, they will under-mine your health. Insulin resistance leads to metabolic syndrome (Syndrome X), obesity and diabetes. Leptin resistance leads to the storing of inessential fats. Cura Romana appears to restore both insulin and leptin sensitivity, which is likely to be one of the reasons it is so successful for weightloss.

The Bottom Line

If Simeons' Roman Cure is indeed delivering on its prom-ises – whether or not we will ever have sufficient, unbiased research to 'prove' this beyond reasonable doubt – what is the fundamental difference between Cura Romana and the weightloss diets which end in frustration for so many who try them? The answer is simple. No other weightloss programme addresses the root cause of obesity. Simeons' Protocol targets *inessential* adipose deposits, enabling the body to restore its natural shape

---

and form. It does *not* burn essential structural fat, nor muscle tissue, the way other diets do. Abnormal hunger disappears on the programme. One no longer has to deal with a sense of deprivation or call on willpower. Cura Romana accomplishes these things by resetting the metabolism via the diencephalon in the brain.

Money Squandered

For more than a decade, the National Institutes of Health in the United States have funded trials to the tune of $150 million in an attempt to discover if 'lifestyle modification' can prevent metabolic syndrome, obesity and adult-onset diabetes. All their trials have been based on conventional 'wisdom' about weight control, most of which is inaccurate. At the moment the NIH are spending $200 million on a long trial which they have named 'Look Ahead'. According to psychologist John Foreyt, one of the trial's investigators, the goal of this research is to test the rather absurd hypothesis that 'overweight diabetics will be healthier if they lose weight'. This, we are told, is 'the largest, most expensive trial ever funded by NIH for obesity outcome research'.

Despite lavish sums of money being spent, such trials will never give us the information needed to affirm what savvy health practitioners and ordinary people know already, thanks to plain old common sense and a bit of time spent digging for truth.

If ever you decide to take time out to plough through the voluminous research and declarations about obesity, its cause and its cure (a pastime I would hardly recommend), you will discover that certain conclusions demand to be drawn:

1 Obesity is not a disorder caused by lack of exercise.

2 Obesity is not caused by over-eating or lack of willpower. It is a state of excess fat accumulation as a

result of some, as yet *officially* unidentified, disequilibrium in the hormonal regulation of fat metabolism. This
is the major issue that must be addressed to conquer
the epidemic of chronic overweight.

3 Because of the effect they exert on insulin and blood
sugar, refined carbohydrates, sugars and starches are
undeniably the dietary culprits in the development of
diabetes, coronary heart disease and obesity. They are
also inevitable contributors to other diseases of civilization, including cancer and Alzheimer's disease.

4 With the exception of chemically distorted oils and
fats full of trans-fatty acids, traditional oils and fats such
as olive oil, coconut oil and butter do not cause obesity.

5 Cereals, grains and sugar-based carbohydrates do.
They distort hormonal regulation and homeostasis,
fostering obesity as a consequence of the way they
disturb insulin balance. They engender insulin resistance syndrome or metabolic syndrome (Syndrome X).

6 Because carbohydrate foods such as these stimulate
insulin secretion, they also increase hunger and diminish
the energy available to the body to fuel good metabolic
processes and for use during day-to-day life.

Track Records

Simeons had successfully treated more than 10,000 people by the time
he died. Swiss surgeon Trudy Voigt reported on 6,000 obese patients
successfully treated with Cura Romana at Bellevue-Klinik in Zurich
over a period of twelve years (*Aesthetic Plastic Surgery*, Vol. 4, pp.
109–15, 1980). She states: 'Daily injections of 125 IU of human
chorionic gonadotrophin, combined with a special 500-calorie diet, has

proven to be a successful medical treatment. It had a rapid effect in reducing body contour circumferences over the full course of treatment and offered the patient a sense of well-being and satisfaction.'

Daniel Oscar Belluscio, MD, in Argentina, has written more extensively than any other physician in the world about Simeons' Protocol, exploring in depth every aspect of Cura Romana and teaching doctors throughout the world how to use it. By 2008 he had successfully treated 14,000 cases of obesity. He continues to do so. Belluscio began his work with Cura Romana using Simeons' original, injectable form of hCG and has since developed an oral form which he now uses. He is director of the Oral hCG Research Centre in Buenos Aires, which disseminates – free of charge – reliable information about the Protocol to doctors worldwide who wish to learn about it.

Together Voigt and Belluscio published a report that is well worth looking at: 'Controversies in Plastic Surgery: Suction-Assisted Lipectomy and the hCG Protocol for Obesity Treatment'. In it they do not advise surgical procedures as the first choice for managing a distorted, overweight body. They report: 'The hCG method for obesity treatment appears to be a complete programme for the management of obesity' (*Aesthetic Plastic Surgery*, Vol. 11, pp. 131–56, 1987). In this published article there are a number of full-colour nude photographs which demonstrate the changes in body shape and form that take place in men and women who have been through the Protocol. Some show the way stretch marks alleviate or disappear. Others record how fat shed from arms and legs has not resulted in sagging skin nor eaten away at muscle mass. All testify to the remarkable re-sculpting of the body that occurs on Cura Romana.

Enough about the important background to Cura Romana. It's time to dive into the practical nitty-gritty. Time to meet the Protocol face to face. Time to get started.

PART TWO

THE
PROTOCOL

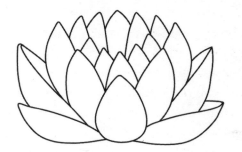

GREAT EXPECTATIONS

'THE TIME HAS COME,' the Walrus said, 'To talk of many things'. Let's take a look at a few fundamentals and answer some important questions: 'What can you look forward to when you begin a Cura Romana Journey?' 'What are its blessings?' 'Its challenges?' 'How do you handle both?' And finally: 'What do you need to be especially clear about?'

In this part of the book – 'The Protocol' – you will learn about these things in my own words. We will also call on former participants of the programme who, having completed their own Cura Romana Journeys, generously offered to share with you some of their experiences – both positive and negative. Aaron and I continue to be grateful for the honesty of their feedback and the support and help they continue to offer other men and women who want to embark on the programme. I always value words 'from the horse's mouth'. I hope you will too.

Ripe for Change

Many who have been drawn to take the Roman Cure Journey tell us that, even before starting the programme, they had a sense of being at a place in their lives where they were itching to discover new relationships with their bodies, their lives and the world around them. I am not sure why, but this is the case. I suspect that when we unconsciously send out this kind of call, a means for fulfilling our desire often presents itself. The way in which participants experience transformation depends upon the needs of their bodies and on the areas of their lives that are ripe for change and growth.

Good News for Vegetarians

Simeons found it impossible to deal with vegetarians on Cura Romana.

Happily, things have changed a lot in the past fifty years. We now have foods – such as micro-filtered whey – which no one in the 1950s even dreamed of. Aaron and I have worked with many vegetarians and find that they do well on Cura Romana. In the process we have discovered some excellent protein alternatives. For vegetarians, the principles of the Food Plan are the same as for the rest of us – four foods per meal and so forth, but using these alternative proteins. Even non-vegetarians tell me they enjoy using these while on hCG+Food Plan. If, even as a vegetarian, you are able to include fish and shellfish in your menus, this is ideal. It gives a lot of variety and fish is an excellent source of easily digested top-quality protein.

Metabolic Rebalancing

Cura Romana's goal is to help the body rebalance its metabolism so that, even after you stop taking the homeopathic, it will go on burning calories efficiently. Together with the diet Protocol, the minute quantities of the homeopathic that you use each day instruct the fat cells – via the hypothalamus – to let go of the fat they hold by turning it into energy. This means that, even while you sleep, your body continues to lose unwanted fat.

Once you complete hCG+Food Plan, your metabolic processes will be in good order. Your body will also have cleared out a lot of collected wastes it had been carrying. You will feel clearer and more balanced physically, mentally and emotionally. These positive results enable you to become aware of two simple yet fundamental keys to health and lasting leanness: how to discover the foods your body 'loves' and thrives on; and how to identify the foods your body 'hates'. The latter will be foods that undermine your health, dampen your spirits, diminish mental clarity and trigger weight gain. Finding out these two things is the purpose and major goal of Consolidation (see Part Three). Once you have done so, you can live your life free of cravings, unnatural hunger and all the worries you once had about weight gain. This will surprise you: once you know these things, you will be able to eat as much as you want of the former and cut out the latter – or eat them only occasionally and in small quantities. Then not only will you not gain weight again, but everything about you will continue to thrive. Why? Because your diencephalon functioning will remain balanced and your weightloss can become permanent.

Better Than a Workout

On the Protocol, your body will be turning somewhere between 1,500 and 4,000 calories per day from fat into energy. Do you have any idea how long you would have to work out to burn even 1,500 calories? You can work out for 4–5 hours a day and never burn that much. The homeopathic hCG+Food Plan directs your metabolism via a signalling pathway in the diencephalon, providing you with the energetic nourishment you would ordinarily expect from eating a huge steak. This is taken from your own fat each day. This helps bring to an end the frustration people experience when trying to lose weight. If you follow the Protocol as it is set out, you not only shed fat efficiently, but you put yourself on a road that can help you experience better health for life.

The diencephalon regulates many of your body's important processes via the autonomic nervous system. In addition to heart rate, breathing, sleep and sexuality, it looks after how well – or how badly – you deal with stress, your energy levels and your spirits. Thanks to the pituitary gland – an important member of the diencephalic group – it helps regulate hormonal balance. The hypothalamus determines the *set point* for your body's weight. Like the thermostat that controls heating in a room, your set point tells your body how much fat it needs in order to ensure survival. Another important goal on hCG+Food Plan is helping your body establish a new, lower set point – a lower weight at which you feel comfortable. One of the jobs during the Consolidation process is consolidating this new set point to help your body make it last.

When you are continually under stress and eating erratically – the way many of us do with our fast-paced lives – your body releases stress hormones like cortisol, telling the hypothalamus to lay down more fat, raise your set point and make you fatter.

Set Point Reset

HCG+Food Plan acts in the brain, resetting the set point for weight and releasing energy from inessential fat stores. In fact, hCG interacts with around fifty different chemicals in the body, including hormones called *adipokines* secreted from the body's fat tissues, leptin and insulin. These chemicals pass signals between the diencephalon and the fat cells, determining when and how to release stored fat and when to add more. On hCG+Food Plan, such interactions bring about changes in your weight set point. Reprogramming your set point in this way provides you with the opportunity during Consolidation to ensure that the reset lasts so that weight-loss can last.

Why We Eat

Hunger signals from the hypothalamus tell us when we want to eat. These signals result from three primary situations:

- When the body is calling for energy, you turn to food in the hope that this will supply it. Sadly, this seldom works. Eating often increases hunger instead of quelling it.
- When the body is in need of a specific essential nutrient – a vitamin or mineral, for instance – or, more often, when it needs a combination of nutrients of which you are not getting enough – this can trigger hunger.
- When experiencing negative emotions or stress, you seek comfort from food – most often cereal and grain-based carbohydrate foods and/or sugar – to which you may have habitually turned for help in the past.

All these triggers are regulated by the hypothalamus and the autonomic nervous system as a whole. Most of them are unconscious. Mostly we are not even aware that they are happening as we reach for food. Conventional weightloss diets use all sorts of techniques in the hope of overcoming such unconscious trigger mechanisms. They ask that you focus on calorie-counting, for instance. They tell you that you must exercise every day. They demand that you use brute force to deny your impulse to eat. As a result, they eventually fail.

Thanks to the way in which hCG+Food Plan enhances the functioning of the hypothalamus and the way the autonomic nervous system behaves, unconscious triggers for eating are gradually cleared away *from inside out*, setting you free of compulsions, self-criticism and food cravings.

Transformation on the Way

While this is going on, other important changes are taking place. Hunger diminishes or disappears. People report feeling better and better as their programme progresses. They no longer have to wrestle with the irritability or weakness common to diets they have done before.

> 'I never felt hungry and please note that I also gave up smoking to start Cura Romana. At that time I had been smoking more than 20 cigarettes a day.'
> *Anna in Italy shed 24 pounds*

Others do experience some hunger during the first few days until the new way of diencephalic function starts to become evident:

> 'I did feel hungry at the start as I had been a grazer. Getting to establish eating times on the programme was my challenge. I quit being hungry in the second week.'
> *Jessie in New Zealand shed 30 pounds*

Food cravings diminish and vanish:

> 'After the first week, I noticed long-standing cravings such as sugar and coffee were leaving me. No more headaches and no bloated stomach. No more acid reflux.'
> *Nilguen in New Zealand shed 24 pounds*

People sleep better. Many find also that they need to sleep less:

> 'I used to wake a couple of times in the night and was not able to get back to sleep. Now I'm able to sleep through. I find I only need about six hours of sleep per night. Instead of feeling sleep-deprived, I wake up ready to get moving for the day.'
> *Christine in Australia shed 22 pounds*

As the system adjusts to its new way of functioning, the body continues to reshape itself. This brings with it a new feeling towards your body as you watch its natural contours being restored:

> 'Inches keep disappearing from my waist, which is great for health. I'm really happy and celebrating this! Had heaps of comments about how I look. They can't believe my "no tummy". I can feel joy and the beginnings of passion where my tummy used to be. I have never felt like this. I feel happy and proud of myself. How bloody fabulous.'
> *Aryana in New Zealand shed 33 pounds*

Such experiences are common to Cura Romana. Each tends to be unique to the individual, because each of us transforms physically, emotionally and spiritually in our own way and at our own speed.

> 'My energy has been high from the word go. I've wanted to get out and do things ... hike, go on walks, enjoy life. It's been amazing.'
> *Megan in South Africa shed 55 pounds*

Not everyone taps into high energy right from the start. Some – I count myself among them – begin the programme carrying what I call a *fatigue deficit*. This is my way of describing an underlying deep fatigue which may have developed as a result of prolonged overwork (in *my* case), chronic stress, yo-yo dieting or drinking. They can experience a few days at the start when they need more rest until the new functioning brought about by the Food Plan and the hCG kicks in. Others experience periods of dynamic energy interspersed with times of fatigue. Both are not only normal but can be enormously important in putting us in touch with the body and its shifting needs from day to day – or sometimes even from hour to hour.

> 'It probably took a good week before I started to tune in with what was happening to my body. I wasn't sure what I needed to do differently and why I didn't have more energy. Leslie's advice was to listen to my body and rest when I needed to.'
> *Mike in New Zealand shed 26.4 pounds*

This is one of the important things you will learn on Cura Romana – how to balance your energies for lasting strength, mental clarity and the kind of fundamental energy that lasts. It makes everything in your life run more smoothly. Most of us still need to learn to honour the body's natural flow between its dynamic outpouring of energy – so exciting, so creative and so much fun – and its *inner-directed*, receptive energy, which, by its nature, is peaceful, sensuous and blissful. The inner-directed state brings us a quiet experience of *being* – of not having to be continually *doing*. It allows us to *receive* what the Universe longs to bring us. We cannot receive its gifts until we know how to move from the dynamic state into the receptive one and back again. When we are tired, the body is asking us to heed the call so that we can restore energy balance. More about this later in 'The Transformation' (see page 322).

Better Health

If you are on any prescription medication it is important that you let your doctor know that you intend to do the Cura Romana programme. If he or she asks for more information about Cura Romana, give him a copy of this book and also the link to Simeons' book *Pounds and Inches*, which is available from www.curaromana.com. The improvements that take place on the programme, as measured by medical parameters, can be significant and rapid. Your doctor will need to check from time to time the dosage of a medication you have been taking. It is likely it will need to be reduced as you progress.

> 'After nineteen years on high-strength thyroid hormone and six years on medication, I am completely off all medication, have never felt better and my blood pressure is naturally lower than it was when I took beta blockers.'
> *Sigrid in Ireland shed 37 pounds*

This is true whether you are on a simple medication for reflux, or a drug for diabetes, high blood pressure, cholesterol control or depression. The improvement that the programme brings about can be dramatic. Your doctor will not want you to continue taking more medication than needed.

> 'My cholesterol dropped by 70 per cent. My irritable bowel symptoms disappeared.'
> *Karen in Australia shed 31 pounds*

> 'I no longer take any Ciprimal or any Zanax. Now I am free of all the medication I was taking and my libido has returned!'
> *Beryl in Ireland shed 6 pounds*

It is *essential* if you suffer from gout, gallstones, diabetes or have recently been treated for a coronary occlusion that your doctor monitors your progress while you are on the programme. These conditions are not contra-indications for Cura Romana, but in such cases the Protocol must be carried out, as Simeons says, *'under the watchful eye of a wise physician'*.

An Exacting Protocol

Your major challenge as you begin Cura Romana is to keep reminding yourself that the diet programme is highly specific. As Simeons says, 'the hCG plus diet method can bring relief to every case of obesity, but the method is not simple.' You really do need to follow it to the letter. To give you an example, a woman on the programme in America was doing great. Her weight was falling away. Then it suddenly stalled, even though she had been very careful about what she was eating and putting on to her body. She couldn't figure out why weightloss stopped. After a lot of questioning, we worked out that a baby had come to stay in her house. She had been smearing nappy cream on its bottom several times a day. Her hands were absorbing the cream and this was preventing further weightloss. Once we identified the problem, she bought some inexpensive plastic gloves which she wore when treating the baby's bottom. Immediately her weightloss resumed.

Another woman on hCG+Food Plan was visiting her parents' home for a few days. She had been washing dishes in water that contained oil and grease from the roasts her parents ate. Her weight stalled. Then she realized her hands had been absorbing oils through her skin. She took to wearing rubber gloves when washing their dishes.

If you have to prepare food for others – for instance, to make a pie crust – buy a packet of thin gloves of the kind surgeons use and always wear them while you're doing this.

Your Way

The physical, spiritual and emotional transformation Cura Romana brings is highly individual. In what ways do you long to transform your own life? Write them down before beginning the programme. Intention, coupled with the Protocol, fuels powerful personal transformation at every level.

Your Cura Romana Journal

Buy yourself a journal. If you already have a notebook you love to write in, great. If not, treat yourself. It needn't be fancy, but it needs to be *special to you*. Make sure it's large enough that you don't feel cramped writing in it. Use it daily to record what you have to eat and drink, how you feel, what worries you, your triumphs and the delights you experience. It's essential that you keep accurate records. Then, when you come up against any kind of challenge – say your weight stalls for more than a day or two – you can check back, identify what could have caused this and work out whether or not you are experiencing a normal pause or if you need to make some kind of change. In another section of your journal, record insights that come to you. There are likely to be many. Later, during Consolidation, you will be recording the experiences you have which help you identify those foods your body loves and those it hates. First, and most important of all, even before you are ready to start your Cura Romana Journey, use your journal to write down your longings, your desires and your intentions for it.

(At the back of this book you will find a section entitled 'Notes', which you can also use to jot down information you might like to record as you're reading through the book.)

Intentions matter

Whether you have as little as 15 pounds to lose, or as much as 100 pounds or more, your key to success is following clear, accurate, easy-to-use information coupled with the best week-by-week guidance system money can buy. Aaron and I spent more than three years creating Leslie Kenton's Cura Romana®. The lion's share of what we have discovered you will find in this book. I can't stress enough how important it is for you to read and re-read it, digesting and absorbing everything in it (no puns intended). The information you will find here can help you experience the best possible Cura Romana Journey in your unique way.

As you wake each morning, and again before you go to sleep at night, get into the habit of saying a short, silent thanks to your body for how well it has served you until now. Then ask it to continue supporting you as your Cura Romana Journey progresses. Tell it that this is a process you have chosen to follow because you want to honour it – to uncover its true form, to nurture it, to strengthen it and to free it from the burden of excess weight.

Intention is a powerful force.

Meanwhile, here is what I intend. It is my intention to share with you the benefits of my experience of Simeons' Protocol, of my work with the hundreds of men and women from all walks of life whom I have mentored on the programme, my knowledge of how it works homeopathically, how to avoid pitfalls, how to make your weightloss last. Most important, I'd like to help you to experience not so much a *new* you as the splendour of the *true* you. That true you is calling you, as it calls from within each one of us. It's asking that you notice its magnificence, see it and help to set it free.

READY STEADY

Let's get down to practicalities. You'll need to gather a few supplies to get ready for the Cura Romana Journey. If you're like me, you'll order them over the internet. Or you can go to a health-food shop, a pharmacy and a good homeware store. For the most up-to-date and best online shopping, check out the resources page at *www.curaromana.com*.

Your Homeopathic

At the top of the list, you will need to order two 15ml bottles of Leslie Kenton's Cura Romana® homeopathic spray (see 'Resources', page 340). You will carry one with you at all times to make sure you have it when you need it while at work or away from home.

Digital Scales

You will need digital bathroom scales to weigh yourself naked every morning as soon as you get up. Only digital scales can give you the accuracy you need. Accuracy is always a primary concern on Cura Romana.

Also, if you don't already own them, buy digital kitchen scales to weigh your protein foods in grams. All the meat and fish you eat must be very carefully weighed raw. You are allowed no more than 100g of fat-free protein at each meal.

You can find good-quality, inexpensive scales of both kinds if you shop around.

Cleansing Support

It is important that your bowels stay reasonably open while you are on the programme. You will be eating very little food, so don't be surprised if you have a bowel movement only every second day or so. I have been surprised to learn that many of the people I've worked with on the programme had suffered with constipation for a long time before starting on Cura Romana. Constipation at any time suppresses energy and can make you feel less than great. You want to avoid it. Get yourself some psyllium seed husks (also called hulls) that have been finely ground to a loose powder. Psyllium – properly called *Plantago asiatica* – has many health benefits. Above all, it's a wonderful source of non-soluble fibre. Each morning you'll use a rounded teaspoonful of it mixed into a large glass of water, say 250ml, and taken with a little stevia (see page 118) if you like. *Do not use more.* Too much psyllium can clog the intestine instead of facilitating bowel movements. Blend your psyllium vigorously – a small hand-held blender is great for this. Drink immediately so that it doesn't have time to gel. Always take fibre with lots of water. *Do not use proprietary products such as Metamucil.* They contain ingredients such as sugars and other chemicals that can seriously interfere with your programme. Just plain, inexpensive psyllium husks in bulk or in capsule form are what to look for. You will need 4–6 capsules a day if you choose to go the capsule route. Always take them with at least 250ml of water.

Natural laxatives

You will also want to find a good laxative herbal tea of which you can drink one cup each morning. Or you can take a natural herbal laxative capsule based on senna or *cascara sagrada*. But read labels carefully – many of these products have additives, such as forms of sugar, which you must avoid.

Day by day you will want to regulate your intake of fibre and laxative tea according to how your bowels are working. Some days you may need them, other days you may not. Occasionally you may find that you will need an extra cup of the tea. Listen to what your body tells you and follow it. You don't want to have diarrhoea. You do want your stools to be light – not too firm or heavy – and somewhat loose. You will begin using your fibre, vitamin C and bowel tea from your very first Feast Day.

Vitamins

The only vitamin that you will use during hCG+Food Plan is vitamin C. You can return to taking other supplements if you wish as soon as you move into Consolidation. Until then, you will need only 3g of vitamin C each morning – 3,000mg. You can choose vitamin C in powder form and mix it with your fibre, and perhaps a little stevia, then blend it quickly for a few seconds and drink it immediately. If you let it sit or don't blend it before it gels, the mixture goes gooey and becomes hard to swallow. If you prefer capsules, take as many as necessary to provide you with 3,000mg (3g) of plain vitamin C each day. *You must read the labels carefully before you buy*. Most vitamin C these days contains artificial sweeteners and other chemicals – including sugar masquerading under some fancy name.

Oils and Stuff

Most people find it hard to believe that fats, oils, creams and ointments put on the body are absorbed through the skin's surface. They will interfere with weight reduction – just as if you had eaten them. There is an incredible sensitivity to even minor increases in nutritional intake while you are on hCG+Food Plan. As a result of your body's reaction to sugars, starches, oils and fats – whether eaten or introduced through the skin's surface – oils of animal and vegetable origin will interfere with the metabolic reset and can stop weightloss. It's essential that you are mindful of everything that goes into your mouth or comes into contact with your skin during hCG+Food Plan.

> **Simeons says:** *Most women find it hard to believe that fats, oils, creams and ointments applied to the skin are absorbed and interfere with weight reduction by hCG just as if they had been eaten. This almost incredible sensitivity to even such very minor increases in nutritional intake is a peculiar feature of the hCG method. For instance, we find that persons who habitually handle organic fats, such as workers in beauty parlours, masseurs, butchers, etc., never show what we consider a satisfactory loss of weight unless they can avoid fat coming into contact with their skin.*

In 1954 Simeons specified that, and I quote, '*No cosmetics other than lipstick, eyebrow pencil and powder may be used*'. Happily, today's skin-care market is quite different to what it was half a century ago. Then, cosmetic products contained a lot of lanolin and vegetable oils. Today there are a number of oil-free products available, including foundations and sunscreens. But you will need to find them, reading every label with care. You probably won't have to replace *all* your regular hygiene and make-up products while on hCG+Food Plan. But go through your collection of personal-care products, work out which might contain animal or vegetable oils and set them aside, knowing that you will be able to resume using them as soon as you enter Consolidation. *Replace them with mineral-based skin care, body care and make-up.*

Mineral oils rule

You'll need a mineral-based lotion or cream to use on your face and body while on hCG+Food Plan. It can be just plain *mineral* oil. You can use baby oil, as it is made from mineral oil. *Anything you use on your face or body while on hCG+Food Plan has to be mineral-based.* The best product we have ever found for skin- and body-moisturizing while on hCG+Food Plan is called QV Lotion. It is not available everywhere in the world, but you can easily buy it online if you live in the UK or continental Europe, Australia or New Zealand. It works a treat. Otherwise, find for yourself a mineral-based lotion with no animal or vegetable elements in it. Ask your pharmacist for help. Tell him it must contain no vegetable fats of any kind and no lanolin. Liquid paraffin is a good choice. It may sound revolting, but it has a good texture and works well. Massage therapists on Cura Romana tell me it is excellent for their work on clients while they themselves are on the programne. They can use it in huge amounts week by week with confidence since it will never interfere with their own or other people's weightloss.

Leslie and Aaron's Favourites

Here are our personal recommendations for the best helper products you can find. They come from our own experience as well as from the feedback we've received from hundreds of men and women who have followed the programme.

Good fibre Psyllium husks (*Plantago asiatica*). You can find them in health-food stores either loose or in capsule form. Do not try to use psyllium seeds whole since they contain fat, which you do not want to take in while on hCG+Food Plan. You will probably need 1 teaspoon a day or 4–8 capsules – not 2 capsules as most of the labels state. Whatever fibre you choose, it *must not contain chemicals, oils or sugar in any form.* The best of the best are Organic India Psyllium Husks. Check *www.curaromana.com* for up-to-date online suppliers.

Senna-based tea To help keep your bowels regular I recommend Smooth Move Tea by Traditional Medicinals, or Get Regular Tea by Yogi Tea, but there are others that will do fine, such as Senna Zest. So will a tea you make for yourself from dried senna leaves. If you want to use tea bags look for a senna-based variety that provides

800–1,100mg of senna *per bag*. You can also take a natural, herbal-based, gentle laxative if you prefer.

Vitamin C The only vitamin you will use while on hCG+Food Plan is ascorbic acid, either as a powder or in capsules – 3g a day. You want either pure ascorbic acid or a buffered vitamin C containing ascorbate forms of the vitamin and *nothing* else. Make sure you do not choose a brand that contains sugar or artificial sweeteners and chemical additives.

Face and Body Lotion QV Skin Lotion by Ego is the best we know of. Second choice? Liquid paraffin – *Paraffinum liquidum BP*. Neutrogena do an oil-free lotion. A note of caution: forget so-called organic cosmetics while you are on hCG+Food Plan. Many people think that because something like, say, Dr Hauschka is a wholesome brand, or some other skincare range is organic, then it is okay to use – but it isn't while you are on hCG+Food Plan. *What you choose has to be mineral-oil based.*

Make-up Jane Iredale Makeup – mineral make-up – is the best in the world. Use it if you possibly can. If you do, I predict you'll come to love it not just when on hCG+Food Plan, but ever after. Her Dream Tint Moisture Tint SPF15, topped off with her Pure Pressed Base Mineral Powder SPF20, is ideal. They give superb covering, contain no nasty chemicals, look beautiful and are a healthy treat for skin. Many women (men too, as it happens, since it looks so natural) whom we have introduced to Jane Iredale come to love it. Check online for where to buy these products in your country. You can, if you prefer, buy one of the cheaper mineral-based lookalikes.

As for mascara, eye pencils, lipstick and the rest, most people find they can get away with using whatever they have become used to without disrupting weightloss. Vaseline is great for dry lips. Use it as often as you want.

Toothpaste Your toothpaste may well list sorbitol as the first ingredient. Sorbitol is a sugar alcohol. It is used in *sugar-free foods,* *gums and mints, which, by the way, you must not use at all while on the programme.* You should never use them at all, even afterwards, as, like those dreadful 'diet' sodas, they can make your body toxic, creating food cravings and addictions in the process. Since your toothpaste will be in your mouth for only a few minutes, however, and you don't swallow it, you can get away with using standard toothpastes – but I would recommend that you avoid using mint-flavoured ones. If you want to be extra careful, as I would, try brushing your teeth with sea salt flakes. It's a great way to strengthen the gums too. If you prefer a good natural toothpaste, Weleda do several, including a salt toothpaste and a calendula toothpaste. You can also use baking soda (bicarbonate of soda).

Deodorants The only deodorant to use on hCG+Food Plan is a crystal deodorant. It comes either in a stick which you rub underneath your arms, or as a spray. You can also use a dusting of plain old baking soda.

Hair-colouring Avoid chemical hair colours if you possibly can while on hCG+Food Plan. Most are toxic and may be absorbed through the scalp. Natural colourings such as henna are okay if you must. But try to get your hair coloured before you begin hCG+Food Plan, or wait until it's finished. You can have your hair coloured when you are on Consolidation.

Sunblocks The best for the face is a simple sunblock such as Jane Iredale's Dream Tint Moisture Tint SPF15, made of minerals. Aveeno Oil-Free Sunscreen is okay. Clinique do an oil-free sunscreen, as do some other manufacturers. Just read labels carefully.

Soaps and cleansers You can use liquid petroleum to take off make-up while on hCG+Food Plan. But for our money, the best cleanser of all is Jane Iredale's Makeup Remover Mitt. She has one for women and another for men. Why is it so good? Because it enables you to clean your face with no need for lotions or soaps. You just wet it in warm water and rub it over your face. It removes make-up fast and easily.

Then you rinse the mitt itself (not your skin) using a little hand soap. Hang it up, and it is ready for the next day. One mitt lasts for years. It is all Aaron and I have used for years. Soaps like Simple Soap, Ivory or Zest, or anything *not enriched with oils and creams* will do fine. So will a liquid wash, like QV Skin Wash by Ego, since it contains no animal or vegetable oils.

Shampoos and conditioners Avoid creamy shampoos and conditioners while on hCG+Food Plan. They can be rich in oils that absorb through the scalp. Use Johnson's Baby Shampoo or a volumizing shampoo such as Volume Boost made by VO5. They are cheap and readily available in supermarkets. John Frieda Luxurious Volume Full Splendor Shampoo is a good choice too, despite its rather portentous name. His Luxurious Volume Full Splendor Conditioner is equally good. Don't leave any conditioner on your hair for more than a minute or two while on hCG+Food Plan. Once you enter Consolidation, you can use whatever you like.

For the most up-to-date online products and suppliers, always check the website, which we are continually updating: *www.curaromana.com*. If you come upon some helper products which you love and find work well, do let us know so we can share them with others.

FEARS AND
TREMBLINGS

WHAT ARE THE COMMON worries that people have when getting ready to start Cura Romana? This is the one I hear most often: 'I know it works for everyone else but I'm sure it won't work for me. Nothing *ever* works for me.' If you find yourself feeling this way, it is not surprising. Cura Romana is as different from conventional weight-loss diets as the proverbial chalk and cheese. It is also very different from any other programme that uses hCG. Unless you know someone who has already done the programme with me, or you've read or listened to the reports from men and women who have completed it, the only way you are going to find out if it works for you is to do it yourself.

End the Struggles

The anxieties some people have before beginning the programme mostly come from their earlier experience of dieting. If you have struggled with your own weight in the past, you probably have four things in common with the rest of us who have been in the same boat:

1 Your metabolic processes are sluggish. Your body does not burn the foods you eat as fuel in the way the body of a lean person does. For you to clear the inessential fat stores which distort body shape and undermine health, low metabolism must be left behind. Cura Romana does this.

2 You are often hungry. Hunger is a genuine physiological response brought about by the body needing more energy. This is not a psychological problem in need of 'controlling'. A larger body requires more fuel to run it. When the hunger/weight-control centre in the brain is functioning optimally, many calories from the foods you eat tend to get stored in the form of inaccessible fat – what Simeons refers to as your fat deposit account. The body is unable to draw upon them for energy. So, even after finishing a meal, you can feel a need for even more food. Thanks to the actions of hCG+Food Plan on the appetite-control centre, hormones and brown-fat deposits, you become able to access this deposit account and turn the fat it contains into energy.

3 You eat when not hungry. Food cravings, frequently described as emotional or compulsive eating, are often treated as though they are fundamentally psychological issues. In truth they are mostly physiological in origin. Cura Romana first diminishes them, then often clears them completely.

4 You worry about losing fat from the wrong places. The programme lets your body steadily shed inches and fat from hips, thighs, bellies and other problem areas.

The Secret Revealed

What is the secret to making these struggles part of your past instead of your future? Simple. *Follow the Protocol to the letter, trust your body and let it happen.* (You must be tired of hearing this from me. I keep repeating it again and again because it is the most important thing about the whole programme and it will make it work for you.) As you do, your body steadily burns fat and begins to shrink in girth. Before long you sense that this body, which, perhaps for years, has been a disappointment to you, is now becoming *your* body in the way it looks and feels. This triggers more changes. Changes in the way you feel about yourself as well as about your life. The changes take place not because of weightloss alone, but because the homeopathic, acting on the diencephalon at the core of the autonomic nervous system, begins gently to lift away from you many unconscious behaviour patterns and limiting beliefs.

> 'Cura Romana has given me back parts of myself that I hadn't connected with for a long time. It's changed old habits and patterns that were keeping me stuck in a state of unhappiness that I'd grown to accept as "normal". With ever-increasing energy, I now confidently embark on the journey of experiencing life instead of watching life happen to me.'
>
> *Rod in the United States shed 33 pounds*

I can't quantify this scientifically, but I see it happen again and again. Participants are continually telling us how patterns continue to clear, thanks to a process which begins on Cura Romana and carries on long after it is finished.

> 'The programme did something that no one and nothing else on this earth could have achieved. It cured me of a cycle of depressive illness that started in 1993 and has prevented me from engaging in life fully ever since. How on earth can you put a price on giving someone's life back.'
> *Karen in England shed 32 pounds*

Ease Your Mind

If you have a history of dieting, you probably know what it's like to feel caught between a rock and a hard place. You may come to fear that any fat you lose is bound to come creeping – or galloping – back as it has before. You worry that you would be unable to cope with the disappointment you've felt before should this happen one more time.

When you were dieting without support from hCG+Food Plan, your body – in an attempt to conserve its energy reserves – tried to wring the last drop of energy from anywhere it could. As it had very little access to inessential fat deposits, it would eat away at your natural, normal fat reserves. In the process it ate away muscle – your protein tissue. This lowered your metabolic rate even further. Then, with each failed diet, it took fewer and fewer calories – which meant smaller quantities of food – for you to regain the weight you lost. It also reduced the number of mitochondria – little factories in muscle cells where fat can be burned as energy. In effect, your whole metabolic chemistry went into *conservation* mode, making it harder and harder to lose weight every time you tried.

When muscle tissue is lost and weight is regained, this not only further diminishes your ability to burn fat but it also depletes your strength and stamina. There are many walking around – especially women – who look 'thin' but carry a very high ratio of fat to muscle in their body as a result of years of yo-yo dieting and food deprivation. They have little vitality, yet they are continually forced to count calories in order to eat less and less to protect themselves from weight gain.

Cura Romana changes this. It helps your body overcome the inertia of weightloss by shifting your metabolic functioning into a dynamic mode where your body is burning stored fat and producing energy. This means that, in time, you no longer have to suffer the kind of energy swings that once had you reaching for something starchy or sweet or relying on coffee to keep going. This can be a different experience than you may have been used to. Some claim this is one of the greatest benefits they get from Cura Romana.

'This is the most rewarding thing I have ever done for myself. It's like striking gold. I sleep deeply, have loads of energy and have transformed my life on so many levels. No words could express what this programme has done for me. I thank God every day that I came across it and have finally won this battle for good.'

Megan in South Africa lost 55 pounds

Unique to You

You may lose weight rapidly in the beginning. Your body may be ripe to let go of a lot of waste that you have been carrying. You may lose more slowly at the beginning and then speed up. Some lose steadily from day to day. If you are one of the fast losers at the beginning of the programme, don't let yourself get cocky and start thinking you can add an extra apple here, a few more grams of protein there and 'get away with it'. You can't.

Everyone on the programme – well, a good 90 per cent anyway –

experiences a few days when their weight stalls. This is a completely normal experience. It is nothing for you to worry about *provided* you just carry on following the Protocol to the letter.

Mysteries of an Empty Fat Cell

Cura Romana turns fat into energy rapidly, leaving the cells in which fat was stored 'empty'. This can cause your weightloss to stall temporarily. Here's how it works. The non-fat contents of the cells from which the fat has been removed and the cell walls require more time – from a few days to a week sometimes – to be broken down. In the meantime, they can fill up with water. It is this which results in temporary stalls. They are of no consequence. Provided you continue to adhere to the Protocol as carefully as ever, the water is lost automatically and your weight begins to drop again in a few days. The important thing to know is that this kind of natural weight stall does not at all interfere with your body's ongoing fat-burning. It just goes on. The mystery is that, even though the scales show little change for a few days, your body continues to lose inches. The gift of all this is that, in his wisdom, Simeons even worked out a simple 'fix' to help you handle natural weight stalls. It's called an Apple Day – see page 129.

In a few people – usually those who have not yet understood how the programme works – a natural weight stall can precipitate a sense of panic: 'Oh my God, what am I doing wrong? Is it all falling apart?' It is important that, throughout Cura Romana, you continually remind yourself that weightloss takes place for each of us in a unique manner. This is determined by your body's own way of directing things. The process you experience on hCG+Food Plan is *your* process. Your body has deep wisdom. Trust that it will take you where you want to go. What you are looking for is an overall weightloss of 0.5– 0.6 pounds a day if you are a woman and an overall weightloss of around a pound a day if you are a man.

> **Simeons says:** *The weight registered by the scale is determined by two processes not necessarily synchronized under the influence of hCG. Fat is being extracted from the cells, in which it is stored in the fatty tissue. When these cells are empty and therefore serve no purpose, the body breaks down the cellular structure and absorbs it, but breaking up of useless cells, connective tissue, blood vessels, etc., may lag behind the process of fat-extraction. When this happens the body appears to replace some of the extracted fat with water which is retained for this purpose. As water is heavier than fat the scales may show no loss of weight, although sufficient fat has actually been consumed to make up for the deficit in the 500-Calorie diet. When such tissue is finally broken down, the water is liberated and there is a sudden flood of urine and a marked loss of weight. This simple interpretation of what is really an extremely complex mechanism is the one we give those patients who want to know why it is that on certain days they do not lose, though they have committed no dietary error.*

The more comfortable you come to feel with the way your weightloss is progressing, the more relaxed you become. As you learn to let go and trust, the whole experience becomes more graceful. It just *happens* while you give thanks to your body for the gifts it is bringing you, look after your day-to-day commitments and watch it all proceed. Before long you are likely to sense that something rather wonderful is taking place and start to think, 'Wow, who would ever have thought that this could happen to me?'

Health-changing

Cura Romana is not only about becoming leaner, it's about encouraging your body to establish better hormonal balance, about slowly building deep strength and vitality – about helping you enhance your well-being all round. As you enter into Consolidation, you begin to discover new ways of eating that are right for *you*. All this, coupled with the simple spiritual practices which you will read about in 'The Transformation' (see page 283), can help you forge a whole new relationship with your body. It can help you renew your metabolic biochemistry, rebalance blood sugar and restore lost insulin sensitivity.

Cura Romana is a truly holistic approach – not only when it comes to fat loss but also in relation to high-level health, good looks and energy. You may be surprised by just how far-reaching the beneficial effects are. Many of the physical improvements it brings can be verified in medically measurable ways.

> **Simeons says:** *In an obese patient suffering from a fairly advanced case of stable diabetes of many years duration in which the blood sugar may range from 300–400 mg, it is often possible to stop all anti-diabetes medication after the first few days of treatment. The blood sugar continues to drop from day to day and often reaches normal values in 2–3 weeks . . . All rheumatic pains, even those associated with demonstrable bony lesions, improve subjectively within a few days of treatment, and often require neither cortisone nor salicylates . . . when an obese patient with an abnormally high cholesterol and already showing signs of arteriosclerosis is treated with hCG, his blood pressure drops.*

On a mundane level, the Roman Cure can make you look and feel younger. It can improve the quality of your skin while building sleek, curved shapes to arms, legs, torso and belly. It helps clear away former feelings of powerlessness and being out of control in relation to food.

By the end of the first week on the programme the body and face often begin to reveal a more toned appearance and feel. By the end of the second week many people sense they are tapping into a new experience of emotional balance. The stresses in life remain but, where they once unsettled you, you now handle them with greater ease.

Homeopathic Secrets

If you are not familiar with homeopathic remedies, you may wonder how our homeopathic hCG works. The homeopathic hCG we formulated and tested for Cura Romana is a safe and stable remedy. It relies on five carefully selected potencies of hCG, some of which carry only its molecular energy. People who have experienced both the homeopathic and the injectable version of the Protocol affirm that there is no difference between them in terms of rapid weightloss. However, the advantages of this homeopathic hCG are many. They include not having to attend a clinic each day for injection, as well as the convenience of being able to carry a bottle of hCG in your pocket or handbag to use while you are out and about. Personally, I believe that the most valuable advantage of this particular homeopathic formula is the sense of spiritual lightness combined with mental, emotional and spiritual well-being that participants report while using it.

No Magic Wand

Cura Romana is not a magic wand. *It can only do its work provided you are willing to work with it by making sure that you follow the Protocol exactly.* This is essential both during the hCG+Food Plan rapid weightloss period and during the six-week Consolidation period. It is the friendly partnership that forms between you and the programme that makes weightloss and all its other bonuses happen. Your body will let go of its inessential fat in the way it decides is best and at its own speed. Women generally shed between 15 and 20 pounds a month. Men can lose between 20 and 30 pounds a month. A few people shed from 8 to 12 pounds during the first week. Whether your own weight-loss is ultra-speedy, slow and steady, or intermittent makes no difference to your success. Abnormal fat deposits diminish. Fat from double chins, pot bellies and thick thighs is sometimes the first to go; sometimes it is the last. Meanwhile, the body continues to rejuvenate itself inside and out.

All You Need Is Within You

It is important that you remember one thing: the power for bringing about the changes in your body and your life for which you long comes from *inside you*. All Cura Romana does is encourage your body to begin re-establishing normality.

> 'I have never been through such a huge transformational process in my life as I've experienced on Leslie Kenton's Cura Romana. I have never felt so connected to life, to my body, to myself. I love it! Love it! Love it!'
> *Jan in New Zealand shed 26.5 pounds*

It may take you a little time to come to trust this and to honour the process of transformation that's being orchestrated from deep within you. As the days and weeks go on, as the partnership you are forming between you and your programme deepens, you can develop a quiet confidence that the path you are on is taking you to where you want to go. As this takes place, something wonderful can occur. You become aware that all the old fear, guilt, confusion and obsession with food has drifted away. A growing sense of freedom has replaced it – freedom just to be who you are and rejoice in this – something impossible to describe until you have experienced it for yourself.

GOOD TO GO

Almost ready to start? Then let's tie up a few loose ends, review the most important things for you to remember and make sure you have all the information you need to go forward with confidence. I'll answer a few last-minute questions you may have – about exercise, how to handle Feast Days, why it's important to drink a lot of water, and the care and feeding of your homeopathic.

A powerful protocol, Cura Romana must never, ever, be undertaken lightly. A simple yet precise tool for rapid, safe, health-giving weightloss, it is unique in the world. It is essential for your success on the programme that you familiarize yourself with all the information in this book. Don't try to skim the chapters and figure it will all be OK. It won't.

> **Simeons says:** *Any patient who thinks he can reduce by taking a few 'shots' and eating less is not only sure to be disappointed but may be heading for serious trouble.*

The Protocol works for men and women of all sizes, shapes and ages so long as they follow it to the letter. Too many have tried to make up new-fangled ways of doing things, only to be disappointed by the results. While the principles and basics of the programme are straightforward, it is easy for someone who is not savvy about what he or she is doing to make inadvertent mistakes that undermine weightloss. This is why I keep urging you to read and re-read these chapters until you come to know the programme like the back of your hand before you get started.

> **Simeons says:** *In treating obesity with the hCG + diet method we are handling what is perhaps the most complex organ in the human body. The diencephalon's functional equilibrium is delicately poised, so that whatever happens in one part has repercussions in others. In obesity this balance is out of kilter and can only be restored if the technique ... is followed implicitly. Even seemingly insignificant deviations, particularly those that at first sight seem to be an improvement, are very liable to produce most disappointing results and even annul the effect completely. For instance, if the diet is increased from 500 to 600 or 700 Calories, the loss of weight is quite unsatisfactory.*

One false belief which I ask you to lay aside from now on is the notion that you have to force yourself to exercise, pushing your body hard, to lose weight and to maintain your weightloss once it has taken place. This notion has been shoved down our throats since the 1980s. It is simply untrue. Don't get me wrong. Exercise is great for health and energy but *only when you do it for the joy of it* – not when you grit your teeth and go to the gym because you think you *must*. During Consolidation and afterwards, I suggest you exercise only out of a love of doing it. Listen to your body. It will tell you what it wants you to do. Follow its wishes and you can't go wrong.

Go Easy

How about exercising while on hCG+Food Plan? If it is easy and fun for you, great, then do it. But take it easy, especially during the first week or ten days. Your body will be entering a period of rapid transformation on every level – from deep cleansing, diencephalic adjustment, rebalancing the autonomic nervous system and hormones to helping you learn to move gracefully from dynamism to a state of quiet relaxation and back again. Give the homeopathic and the Food Plan a chance to do their work. Vigorous, strenuous exercise early on in the Protocol can divert the body's attention from the task at hand.

By all means go for a 30-minute walk once a day – preferably in a park, under trees or in the country if you can. Walking for pleasure is excellent while on hCG+Food Plan. It supports the development of a new relationship between you and your body, as well as your physical and spiritual transformation. You can also swim gently if you love the water. Or do relaxing yoga. You might try a little gentle bouncing on a mini-trampoline. Once you enter Consolidation, there will be time enough to increase your exercise while you are expanding your food choices.

Simeons allowed only those patients who adored exercise and were used to doing it regularly before Cura Romana to exercise while weightloss was taking place. He also spoke about an interesting phenomenon that can be experienced by a few people at the end of Cura Romana.

Simeons says: *Towards the end of a full course when a good deal of fat has been rapidly lost, some patients complain that lifting a weight or climbing stairs requires a greater muscular effort than before. They feel neither breathless-ness nor exhaustion but simply that their muscles have to* *work harder. This phenomenon, which disappears soon after the end of the treatment, is caused by the removal of abnormal fat deposited between, in and around the muscles. The removal of this fat makes the muscles too long, and so in order to achieve a certain skeletal movement, say the bending of an arm, the muscles have to perform greater contraction than before. Within a short while the muscle adjusts itself perfectly to the new situation, but under hCG the loss of fat is so rapid that this adjustment cannot keep up with it. Patients often have to be reassured that this does not mean that they are 'getting weak'. This phenomenon does not occur in patients who regularly take vigorous exercise and continue to do so during treatment.*

Water, Water Everywhere

The control centre for both thirst and hunger is in the diencephalon. Often when you think you are hungry what your body is trying to tell you is that you need to take in more water. One of the best-kept secrets in the world about weight control is this: reach for a glass of water every time you feel hungry. You are likely to find your hunger diminishes within 10 minutes.

There is another way in which taking in optimal quantities of water plays a central role in fat loss and weight control. It has to do with your kidneys. The kidneys are responsible for recycling all the water in your body – some 800 glasses of it a day – and for filtering out any wastes present before they can lower immunity, create fatigue or make you feel hungry, even though you may have had enough to eat. These wastes cause the kind of water-retention that plagues so many who have gone on and off slimming diets for years. The filtering mechanism in the kidneys is made up of millions of microscopic bodies known as *glomeruli*. These identify waste products, such as urea, which need to be removed, as well as screening out other chemicals, such as unwanted metals and any excess minerals. Meanwhile, they pour back into the bloodstream the minerals you need and regulate your body's acid–alkaline balance. Ironically, if you tend to retain water, you need to drink more.

> **Simeons says:** *Patients are usually hard to convince that the amount of water they retain has nothing to do with the amount of water they drink. When the body is forced to retain water, it will do this at all costs. If the fluid intake is insufficient to provide all the water required, the body withholds water from the kidneys and the urine becomes scanty and highly concentrated, imposing a certain strain on the kidneys. If that is insufficient, excessive water will be withdrawn from the intestinal tract, with the result that the feces become hard and dry. On the other hand if a patient drinks more than his body requires, the surplus is promptly and easily eliminated. Trying to prevent the body from retaining water by drinking less is therefore not only futile but even harmful.*

Energy-balancing

There is more to the power of water on Cura Romana than just drinking it. You will discover this yourself when you get into Epsom salts baths. These are useful if you are having a stressful day and for deep-cleansing the body both physiologically and energetically. They are ideal for encouraging deep, restful sleep and relaxation.

Epsom salts are magnesium sulphate. Both the magnesium and the sulphate molecules have the ability to leach excess sodium, phosphorous and nitrogenous wastes from the body. As they reduce toxicity, more of the body's energetic potential gets freed up for use. Magnesium and sulphur also happen to be among the most alkalinizing earth minerals. In practical terms, what this means is that they have the ability to create more physical space between the atoms and molecules of your body. The greater the acidity in the body and the more compressed this molecular space becomes, the greater the physical and emotional pressure you feel.

There's more good news. When you step into an Epsom salts bath, the magnesium sulphate immerses your body in a unified electrical field. This takes excess electrical discharge from one area of the body and sends it to areas that are undercharged, creating an energetic balance and flow. There is nothing quite as good as an Epsom salts bath, for instance, when you have been on a long flight or if you are suffering from jet lag, emotional tension or fatigue. But there is a very specific way of taking an Epsom salts bath.

Here's How

Pour 454g industrial-grade Epsom salts into the bath. You can find them at the chemist and in supermarkets, or order them in bulk, cheaply, over the internet. Fill the bath with water at blood temperature (38°C – just above body temperature). Immerse yourself in it for at least 20 minutes. If your body gets too cool, then add some more hot. If your body becomes too warm, add some cold water, so that you are able to sustain being in this bath in a very relaxed state for 20–30 minutes. Then get out of the bath and wrap yourself in a towel.

If you are doing this just before going to bed, climb into bed, cover yourself up, keep warm and you can easily drift into blissful sleep. If it's during the day, or if you are trying to restore yourself to be able to go out in the evening, then when you get out of the bath wrap yourself in a towel and lie down for 10 minutes. Then get up, get dressed and go about whatever you are intending to do.

Participants on Cura Romana find Epsom salts baths are not just useful but an enormous pleasure. If you have any difficulties, particularly in the first week or so when your body is making its powerful transition, Epsom salts baths are great for making it all easier. I find they are always good to keep on hand.

Homeopathic Mysteries

Your Cura Romana homeopathic hCG is one of the newer combination homeopathic products. It has been uniquely and carefully formulated in the UK specifically for the programme, using water plus a small quantity of carefully selected alcohol as a medium for delivering its benefits. The polymorphic structure of the water and alcohol become 'imprinted' by the energetic frequencies of hCG, enabling it to hold and transfer this information to the body.

Physics is probably best suited to an attempt to explain the mysterious mechanics of homeopathy and the energetics behind the activity of homeopathic remedies. It is now known, for instance, that homeopathic remedies emit distinct, measurable electromagnetic signals, and that manufacturing alters the physical geometry of the water-plus-alcohol solute. Science has finally begun developing objective ways of measuring some of the mechanisms by which homeopathic therapeutics carry out their work. Many of these subtle changes can now be observed, thanks to highly sensitive tests using techniques with long, complicated names like nuclear magnetic resonance and Raman-laser spectroscopy.

What's important for you to know is that your Cura Romana homeopathic should be *succussed* to activate it before use. Here's how. Tap the bottle firmly 10–15 times against the heel of your hand before spraying it under your tongue. Then let the liquid sit in your mouth for 10–15 seconds before swallowing. Be sure you carry a bottle of your homeopathic with you at all times so that you can use it when you are away from home.

When you take your homeopathic regularly and consistently, this sends clear, ongoing information to the diencephalon, altering hunger perception, triggering fat-burning, supporting your weightloss and your body as a whole, all the way through the programme and beyond – provided, of course, that you also follow the nine-week dietary Protocol carefully. The amount of homeopathic you will be using, by the way, is the same for everyone. It has nothing to do with your size, your weight, your gender or your age.

Simeons says: *The diencephalon is an extremely robust organ in spite of its unbelievable intricacy. From an evolutionary point of view it is one of the oldest organs in our body and its evolutionary history dates back more than 500 million years. This has rendered it extraordinarily adaptable to all natural exigencies, and that is one of the main reasons why the human species was able to evolve. What its evolution did not prepare it for were the conditions to which human culture and civilization now expose it.*

The Big Day Approaches

From the first morning of your first Feast Day, you will be taking 2 sprays of your homeopathic four times a day. You will continue to take 2 sprays four times a day all the way through to Day 21. Take them first thing, 15 minutes before lunch, 15 minutes before dinner and then again at bedtime. You must get the homeopathic into your system so that on the *third* day of Cura Romana (which will be the *first* day of your hCG+Food Plan) it can begin to do its work.

Also, on the first of your Feast Days, be sure to record your weight first thing in the morning. From your first Feast Day onwards you will weigh yourself naked every morning – as soon as you wake up, after you have urinated. *Never weigh at any other time of the day and never weigh yourself more than once a day.* Always use the same scales. Scales vary tremendously from one to another. If ever you have to be away from home, always take your scales with you.

Your Feast Days are vitally important. They prepare your system to make the transition to hCG+Food Plan with relative ease. Go for delicious, rich foods that you love and make sure they are always good quality. Don't eat junk food. You don't *ever* want to put junk into your system. Choose good-quality ice cream or chocolate. You can have wine if you like. Have pancakes with maple syrup or a good-quality hamburger. Do not worry about gaining weight. The weight you gain on these two days will be lost very, very rapidly. Let yourself enjoy the sensuous pleasure of eating rich, sweet, delicious food. Good Feast Days significantly empower weightloss physiologically. Simeons knew what he was doing. People who don't feast well have a more difficult time in the first days on hCG+Food Plan. So enjoy yourself.

> **Simeons says:** *Most patients who have been struggling with diets for years and know how rapidly they gain if they let themselves go are very hard to convince of the absolute necessity of gorging for at least two days, and yet this must be insisted upon categorically if the further course of treatment is to run smoothly . . . In any case, the whole gain is usually lost in the first 48 hours of dieting. It is necessary to proceed in this manner because the gain re-stocks the depleted normal reserves, whereas the subsequent loss is from the abnormal deposits only.*

A Quiet Word . . .

Focus on where you are going. Give thanks to your body right now – before you begin – for having supported you so well until this day. I'm quite serious. Explain to your body, either out loud or silently in a meditative state, that you have chosen to do your Cura Romana Journey to help it transform itself into its true form, bringing greater strength, vitality and joy.

Let the Transformation Begin

If you are going to experience any week of Cura Romana as challenging, it's likely to be this week – your first week on hCG+Food Plan, just after completing your Feast Days. Many people have no hunger right from the beginning. Others have hunger on and off for the first few days. If you happen to be one of these, don't worry. This will settle down as your body moves into the new, metabolically dynamic state – and all this begins to take place from your very first day on the Food Plan.

Let yourself become aware of how you feel day by day. *If you're tired – rest*. Give your body and psyche a chance to begin their transformations. They can be profound. If, on the other hand, you have masses of energy, enjoy it. If you experience any kind of detox reaction – a headache, for instance, as wastes stored in your body begin to be cleared – take a couple of aspirin or some other kind of painkiller. (If you can, try to 'celebrate' the headaches you might experience, for this is an indication that you are ridding your body of unwanted, unhealthy wastes.) Give yourself some extra time to do something pleasurable. Listen to music, maybe. Or simply lie down. Remember you are now at the beginning of a remarkable journey.

Hungry at the Start

Fifty or 60 per cent of men and women on Cura Romana find that they are not hungry right from the very first day. Well, hopefully they are a little bit hungry before lunch and dinner each day, because that's quite normal. But as far as the real hunger that most people experience on any sort of weightloss programme goes, for most people this is not part of Cura Romana during the first week, nor in fact all the way through.

About 40 per cent of people do feel hunger in the beginning. This is because the body is moving into a very dynamic transformation in the way it feels and functions. Whether or not you feel some hunger for the first few days has no bearing on the success of your programme. Just know that this too will pass when your body has adjusted to its new way of functioning and the remnants of any food cravings you may have had before you started clear from your system.

Often when we think we're hungry what we're really feeling is tired, or we're simply in need of a drink of water. This is something I discovered for myself. Sooner or later, most men and women make the same discovery during their own Cura Romana Journey. What many of us have done in the past when we're weary or anxious is reach for food instead of taking a break. In a way this is a natural thing to do. The trouble is that mistaking the body's longing for rest and eating instead never works. Worse than that, eating when we are tired only further lowers our vitality. Here are some sample actions you can take to quell any feelings of hunger at the beginning of the programme:

1 Try spending 5 minutes paying attention to the way your breath feels as it moves in and out.

2 Go for a short walk.

3 Drink water or herbal tea.

4 Sit down with your eyes closed for a minute or two. Put on some earphones and listen to uplifting music or inspirational words on an MP3 player.

5 Remember what you have chosen to do on Cura Romana is to enter into a journey of total transformation on every level – your energy, your health, your emotional life, your spiritual life and, of course, permanent weightloss.

6 Be patient with your body. Listen to the messages it is trying to give you. The body is always calling to us. Our challenge is learning to hear its whispers as well as its shouts.

What is your body asking from you now? That you rest? That you do something that brings you pleasure apart from eating? That you hang in there until your hunger passes? Ask it. I mean this quite literally. Say it either out loud or quietly from within. You have requested of your body that it help you change its size and shape, enhance its health, increase its vitality and re-establish better balance in other areas of your life. Day by day, speak to your body and find out how you can fulfil its needs too. The partnership that develops between your mind and your body when you do this can be nothing less than life-transforming; it's a partnership that should be nurtured and respected.

The Time Is Now

As you begin your programme, this is the ideal time to start putting behind you any anger or sadness or disappointment that you've felt with your body in the past for its not being what you thought it should be. In the next nine weeks you and your body will be able to get to know each other better than ever before – to become good friends, supporting each other in wonderful, effective ways. Together you can celebrate the changes that are to come.

We are living in a time of deep transformation, not only for ourselves as humans but for the planet as a whole. Poised at the threshold of a remarkable birth process, we can discover new ways of thinking, being and living. Aaron and I, along with a great many participants on the programme, sense that the simple yet profound homeopathic Cura Romana Journey may offer even greater rewards than health-giving, potentially permanent weightloss than we have yet recognized. It can certainly further the process by which each of us becomes more fully the person who, in essence, we already are. As this happens, we not only enrich our own lives and the lives of others, but we contribute to the welfare of our planet as it calls out for a new birth.

The All-important Reset

The goal of your Cura Romana Journey is to help your body reset its metabolism permanently. Your homeopathic uses the brain's hormone-signalling pathways to alter hunger perception and induce rapid weightloss. This brings many other benefits in its wake, because the diencephalon sits at the core of the autonomic nervous system. This remarkable process takes time. As you continue on the dietary programme, using your homeopathic consistently, it makes good connections with the receptors and teaches them new ways of functioning. During hCG+Food Plan, you will be living to a far greater extent on the fat that you are losing than on what you eat. Thanks to the action of the homeopathic coupled with the Food Plan, you are able to draw the extra calories you need from your body's own, inessential fat stores. This is the reason that people on the programme experience little or no hunger.

Good to Go Checklist

Are you ready to begin your Cura Romana Journey? Work through this checklist to make sure you are **Good to Go**:

Tick Box

I have read through the book thoroughly and marked the important things for me to remember in the margins or in my notebook.
This is important. Always go back to the book. Never rely on thinking 'I know all that already.' You will need to refer to it daily. The Protocol is exacting. You want it to work smoothly and gracefully, all the way through.

I have a notebook or journal in which to record each day all my food and drink, my weight, my experiences, my questions and my concerns, as well as my triumphs and any setbacks.
It is essential that you commit yourself to keeping these records day by day to ensure your success all the way through hCG+Food Plan, as well as Consolidation.

I have my hCG spray, and I always carry one bottle with me when I'm out so I can be sure to take it on time. ☐

I know how to succuss homeopathics. I know that I need to take my homeopathic first thing on rising before brushing my teeth, then 15 minutes before each of my two meals, and just before going to bed. ☐
Avoid mint-flavoured toothpaste as it can interfere with your homeopathic.

I have digital scales to weigh myself naked at the same time every morning – starting from my first Feast Day throughout the whole nine weeks. I am committed to recording my weight each day. ☐
If you have to travel during either hCG+Food Plan or Consolidation, take your scales with you.

I have digital scales to weigh my protein foods raw before cooking. ☐

I have my fibre and vitamin C to hand and a way of blending them with 180–240ml water. I intend to take 3g of vitamin C a day, either as powder or in capsule form (see pages 74 and 77 for details on vitamin C). ☐

I have my laxative tea, such as Smooth Move by Traditional Medicinals, or whatever capsules or senna tea I have chosen to use during hCG+Food Plan (see page 76 for details on fibre). ☐

I know how to check in online at www.curaromana.com for the latest information about the programme or for help in locating useful products. ☐

*I have a means of charting my weightloss daily and, if I wish, □
recording my loss of inches once a week.*

I have organic stevia – if I decide to use it. □
You may not use any artificial sweeteners as they are chemically based and can slow weightloss. They are also not good
for your health. **Under no circumstances are you allowed to
use 'diet colas' or sugar-free gum or any other such products on Cura Romana.**

I have Epsom salts at the ready for my relaxing baths. □

I have QV Lotion or some other mineral-based lotion or liquid □
*paraffin to use on my face and body and as a moisturizer
while on hCG+Food Plan.*
QV is a perfume-free, colour-free, propylene glycol-free,
mineral-based lotion for the face and body that does not
interfere with the Protocol. There are other similar lotions
that are entirely mineral-oil-based – see pages 75–76 for
details. Ask a pharmacist or check the label carefully. **Do not
use any oils or creams that are not mineral-based during
hCG+Food Plan, or any products that contain vegetable
oils or lanolin.**

Trust Your Body

When you begin Cura Romana, you enter into a powerful transformational process. Let your body direct the letting-go of your excess weight. There is tremendous wisdom in the body – trust it. Too often we forget this and think we have to use our will. Every part of the Cura Romana Journey proceeds more gracefully if you stop trying to will it to happen. Trust the process. Enjoy the ride. The answer to the question 'How can I manage on 500 calories a day when on hCG+Food Plan?' is this: you can manage very well indeed, without willpower, holding your breath, gritting your teeth or hoping against hope it will happen. It simply does.

So let's begin . . .

LESLIE KENTON'S
CURA ROMANA®
HCG+FOOD PLAN

CURA ROMANA'S nine-week programme is one of transformation for body, mind and spirit and, as I mentioned in Part One, it consists of two parts: the 24-day hCG+Food Plan period – which includes two Feast Days – followed by the six-week Consolidation period. So let's begin with the Feast Days and look at exactly what you will do at the start of your Cura Romana Journey.

YOUR DAILY SCHEDULE
Days 1 and 2: Feast Days

Feast Days are essential. This is when you will build up stores of glycogen and fat so that the three weeks of rapid weightloss happen as smoothly as possible. This is also when you will begin to use your homeopathic spray, as detailed below. Any weight you gain during these two days will be lost in a day or two when you are on the hCG+Food Plan. The small gain re-stocks any depleted normal reserves. Subsequent fat loss then comes only from the abnormal fat deposits.

On rising Weigh yourself after urinating. It is important to weigh yourself naked each morning – not at any other time of day – always using the same scales.

Take your first dose of hCG homeopathic spray – 2 sprays under the tongue, hold for 15 seconds before swallowing. Make sure your mouth is clean for 15–20 minutes before taking your hCG spray. Do not use toothpaste before using it. Wait 15–20 minutes after taking it before doing anything else orally (e.g. cleaning teeth).

Before lunch 15–20 minutes before lunch take your second dose of hCG homeopathic spray: 2 sprays as before. Wait 15–20 minutes after taking your spray before eating lunch.

Before dinner 15–20 minutes before dinner take your third dose of hCG homeopathic spray: 2 sprays as before. Wait 15–20 minutes after taking your spray before eating dinner.

Before bed Take your fourth dose of hCG homeopathic spray – 2 sprays as before.

SPECIAL NOTE ON COFFEE *If having coffee at any time, wait for one hour before or after taking your Cura Romana homeopathic spray.*

SAMPLE FEAST DAY MENU

The following is only an example of a menu for Days 1 and 2 – not a menu for you to follow exactly. There is no need to stuff yourself on your Feast Days. Just enjoy foods containing good, healthy fats, like butter, cream, olive oil and delicious sweet things, including good-quality chocolate. Stay away from packaged junk foods.

Begin taking your homeopathic hCG spray on your first Feast Day (see page 107).

BREAKFAST Cheese omelette, sausages or bacon, or pancakes with maple syrup.

MID-MORNING SNACK Muffin with whipped cream and jam.

LUNCH Lamb chop, baked potato with sour cream and chives, vegetables with melted butter.

MID-AFTERNOON SNACK Ice cream.

DINNER Pasta in sauce sprinkled with Parmesan cheese, salad dressed in olive oil, crème brûlée for dessert.

LATE-NIGHT SNACK Good quality chocolate.

YOUR DAILY SCHEDULE
Days 3–24

Following your two Feast Days, you will begin the Cura Romana Food Plan. You will continue to use your hCG homeopathic spray, as before, 4 times each day, and will weigh yourself, as before, each morning. Below is an outline of what you will do during the hcG+Food period:

On rising Take your first dose of Cura Romana homeopathic spray – 2 sprays under the tongue, hold for 15 seconds before swallowing. Wait 15–20 minutes after taking before doing anything else orally, e.g. cleaning teeth.

Prepare fibre with vitamin C in a blender with 180–240ml water – add stevia if needed. Blend and drink immediately while still liquid – ideally within 60 seconds of blending, otherwise it gels and is quite unpleasant to drink. If you prefer, you can use psyllium husk capsules. You are likely to need 4–6 capsules each morning. Be sure to swallow with lots of water. You can also use pure ascorbic acid in 1,000mg capsules if you prefer – 3 a day.

Have a cup or half a cup of Get Regular by Yogi Tea, Smooth Move by Traditional Medicinals or another senna-based tea, preferably containing 800–1,100mg senna per sachet, or your senna capsules.

> NOTE *Make sure your mouth is clean for 15–20 minutes before taking your hCG spray. Take it on rising. Do not use toothpaste before using your spray.*

Before lunch 15–20 minutes before lunch take your second dose of the hCG spray – 2 sprays as before, hold for 15 seconds. Wait 15–20 minutes after taking your spray before eating lunch.

> NOTE *Have lunch early if you possibly can – experiment to find the right time for you (usually somewhere between 11.30 and 1 p.m.). You want to eat your meals as regularly as possible on hCG+Food Plan. (See pages 122–5 for a full list of the foods allowed, and page 112 for sample menus you can use during this three-week period.)*

Before dinner 15–20 minutes before dinner take your third dose of the homeopathic spray – 2 sprays as before. Wait 15–20 minutes after taking your spray before eating dinner.

> NOTE *It is helpful to have dinner early, if possible – say between 5 and 6 p.m. See pages 122–5 for a full list of the foods allowed, and page 112 for sample menus you can use during this three-week period.*

Before bed Take your fourth dose of Cura Romana homeopathic spray – 2 sprays as before.

> SPECIAL NOTE ON COFFEE *If having coffee at any time, wait for one hour before or after taking your homeopathic spray.*

HCG+Food Choices

During the hcG+Food Plan period, from Days 3–24, you will eat two main meals a day. During this time you will eat no more than 500 calories a day and the way these calories are made up is of enormous importance. For example, if you leave out an apple and eat an extra breadstick instead, although you won't be taking in more calories, this can interfere with weightloss. There are many foods, such as pimento, okra, artichokes and pears, which have the same or even lower caloric values than the foods allowed on the programme, yet they would interfere with the consistent loss of weight.

> IMPORTANT NOTE *on cup measures given here relating to vegetable servings: Vegetables do not need to be weighed in the conventional way. You should aim to fill a standard mug (think 'builder's tea') and pack it to the brim with your vegetables.*
>
> *Do not use this cup measure for fruits, including tomatoes, which are very high in fruit sugar. Fruit and other dry ingredients should be weighed in the conventional way following the quantities given in each recipe.*

Here is a sample of the kind of foods you can choose to eat at each of these two main meals, but please also see pages 122–5 for a full list of the foods allowed, sample recipes and lists of spices, condiments, etc., that you will be able to use to prepare your meals.

- 100g of protein at each meal, chosen from: lean beef and lamb, chicken breast (with skin removed), rabbit, hare, veal, fresh wild white fish, lobster, crab, prawns, shrimps. (Don't eat the same protein twice in one day.)

- One type of vegetable at each meal, chosen from: spinach, Swiss chard or silver beet, chicory, salad greens of any kind, tomatoes, celery, fennel, onions, radishes, cucumbers, asparagus, cabbage. (Don't eat the same vegetable twice in one day.)

- One Italian breadstick (*grissino*).

- One piece of fruit at each meal, chosen from: apple or orange (medium-sized), half a grapefruit or a handful of organic strawberries. (Don't eat the same fruit twice in one day.)

IMPORTANT: Foods, chemicals and other things you should avoid during the hCG+Food period:

Coffee (more than one cup a day), raw garlic and raw onions, very strong spices, mint (including toothpaste), camphor (found in muscle and joint rubs, mothballs, etc.), strong smells (such as paint-thinners, eucalyptus and cigarettes/cigars), hair-colouring. Keep your hCG spray away from sunlight, electronic equipment and X-rays, and do not refrigerate.

NOTE *You are allowed two fruits and two grissini/breadsticks each day. You can eat these fruits or breads as snacks instead of eating them at mealtimes if you prefer.*

SAMPLE HCG + FOOD PLAN MENUS
(Days 3–24)

MENU 1 _____

BREAKFAST

Tea or herbal tea

1 tablespoon milk

LUNCH

100g (weighed raw) skinless chicken breast

1 cup asparagus

1 medium-sized apple

1 grissino/breadstick

DINNER

100g (weighed raw) beefsteak, all visible fat removed

2 cups spinach

8–10 strawberries

1 grissino/breadstick

MENU 2 _____

BREAKFAST

Tea or herbal tea

1 tablespoon milk

LUNCH

100g tinned tuna in spring water or brine

Coleslaw (cabbage with lemon or vinegar, water and herb dressing)

1 medium-sized apple

1 grissino/breadstick

DINNER

100g (weighed raw) grilled venison, all visible fat removed

Rocket, with apple cider vinegar, water and herb dressing

1 medium-sized orange

1 grissino/breadstick

Walking the Talk

Any deviation in foods or in the amounts you are eating (any increase in your caloric intake or any animal or vegetable fat, or oily substances that contact your skin) only creates confusion in the signalling pathway that is in the process of resetting the diencephalon. This can also slow weightloss or even stop it. If these things were to happen frequently, the shift to resetting the way the hypothalamus functions would cease. Then you would find yourself hungry and fatigued as though you were following a starvation diet. This is something you never want to experience.

The Cura Romana Kitchen

Welcome to our Cura Romana, homeopathic hCG+Food Plan kitchen. One of the surprising things about the rapid weightloss portion of Cura Romana is that – once you get used to hCG+Food Plan – you are likely to find that food never tasted better. Personally, I am lazy. I love doing everything as simply and quickly as I can. I go for delicious organic vegetables, fruits – many picked from my own garden – and fresh protein foods. These I often cook in an electric steamer in as little as 15 or 20 minutes. Then, at the same time as I am cooking my chicken, meat or fish, I can also cook my vegetables, say broccoli or spinach. Electric steamers have different levels, enabling you to cook a lot all at once – see page 115. You can even prepare a fruit for dessert at the same time – say an apple sweetened with stevia with some cinnamon sprinkled on top. Otherwise, more often than not, I eat my fruits and vegetables raw. I even eat a lot of sashimi – that is raw fish – on the hCG+Food Plan, but only if it's clean, fresh fish from good waters. I adore raw foods. And, like most people, I thrive on them.

One vegetable per meal

Simeons insisted that you eat only one vegetable at each meal. I insist that everyone do this *for the first ten days on hCG+Food Plan.* Then, provided your weightloss is progressing well, you can *try* mixing a couple of vegetables at the same meal *once a day. Always keep to the same overall quantity of total vegetables that the Protocol allows.* This slight deviation from Simeons' original plan works fine for some. For others, it does not work. Try it, but if you find that your weight stalls, return to having only one vegetable per meal.

First principles: weigh it – measure it

Make sure you have digital kitchen scales that weigh in grams. If you're used to ounces, now is the time to switch over. 100g is approximately 3 1/2 oz. Most modern digital scales convert between ounces and grams at the push of a button. Meat, chicken and fish must always be weighed *raw, skinless and with every trace of fat or shells removed before weighing.* For vegetables (not fruits) please use your 'builder's mug' and pack your vegetables to the brim, as outlined earlier – see page 110.

Buy the best

Go organic if you possibly can. If not – don't get neurotic about it. Just buy the best foods you can afford. Choose meat from grass-fed, free-range animals that are certified hormone- and antibiotic-free. Fresh, wild fish is a great blessing on the programme, as are free-range or organic chicken breasts.

Cooking without oils

Cura Romana strictly excludes the use of oils for cooking and in food. This means you must use methods other than ordinary frying and sautéeing. You can 'dry-fry' proteins on a little salt placed in the bottom of a heavy pan. You can sauté with water in a similar way. You can also use a George Foreman grill, which cuts down on fat and has a non-stick surface. Long-term use of non-stick pans is not a good practice, since this has been linked to health problems; however, you are on hCG+Food Plan for only three weeks. So, if you want to use them, go ahead.

Bake, grill or steam

You can bake or grill your meat and fish. Then there is the wonderful electric steamer. I got mine from one of those silly 'points programmes'. When it arrived I took one look at it and decided it was a piece of junk that I should throw away. Then I tried it once and realized it was good for Cura Romana. It has four layers. In the container which sits on the bottom layer is a little dish perfect for cooking 100g of chicken, fish or meat. Put your vegetables – spinach, Swiss chard/silver beet or asparagus – on the next layer up. Set the timer to 15–20 minutes. Juice from the vegetables drips down to season the meat or chicken, adding flavour. I love the way you can just push a button and 20 minutes later have a meal prepared. Steamers are also useful for cooking family meals long after hCG+Food Plan.

Finally, a piece of equipment that I adore is a blender. Use one on hCG+Food Plan to make a healthful green smoothie. It's also great for making fruit and vegetable smoothies when you are in Consolidation, and for the rest of your life.

No artificial sweeteners

All artificial sweeteners are prohibited. Avoid them like the plague, not only while you are on the programme but for the rest of your life. These include aspartame (Nutrasweet), which is the most toxic of the lot, sucralose (Splenda) and saccharine. Only stevia is allowed for sweetening (see page 118).

No animal or vegetable fats or oils

No fat in your foods, no oils on your skin (except mineral oils), no extra foods – not even a small increase in caloric intake – are allowed while on the hCG+Food Plan. Any deviation in foods or in the amounts you are eating, any increase in your caloric intake, or any animal or vegetable fat or oily substances that contact your skin only create confusion in the signalling pathway which is in the process of resetting metabolism. These things will slow weightloss or stop it. If they were to happen frequently, the resetting process would cease.

The gen on flavourings

Steer clear of common manufactured sauces, even if they say 'low calorie' on the label. Mayonnaise, ketchups, salad dressings and the rest often contain sugar, cornflour and other carbohydrates or oil. You absolutely must not use these on the Protocol. Avoid food additives of any kind like the plague. One of the worst is MSG (monosodium glutamate). Not only does it undermine health in serious ways, it also causes weight gain. The multinational food industry uses it everywhere and it's usually hidden on food labels under various disguises such as 'autolyzed yeast', 'sodium caseinate', 'soy sauce'. It is added to scores of products seen on supermarket shelves. Stay away from them. Similarly, steer clear of low-calorie salad dressings. They can easily interfere with your programme.

Spice it up

While you are on hCG+Food Plan, flavour is everything. Protein foods themselves are always in need of herbs and spices. Don't hesitate to use them. Be creative. Just because a recipe calls for oregano does not mean that it might not be even better if you substitute dill weed. Play with it. The more variety you can get with herbs and spices, the more exciting the foods you prepare will become.

The Cura Romana Protocol permits herbs and spices in unlimited quantities, but it's very important that you check on the quality that you are using. Most of the stuff that's sold in supermarkets has a lot of additives in it, including – believe it or not – sugar, and you don't want additives (you will not find these listed on labels). I would always go for organic herbs and spices.

You can use garlic, no problem, but the garlic is best cooked. Why? Because you are using a homeopathic and homeopathics can sometimes be interfered with by garlic if it's taken raw. If you use raw garlic, give yourself an hour before you take your homeopathic.

Great Herbs and Spices to Choose From

allspice	dill	parsley
angelica	fennel	pepper– black,
basil	fenugreek	white and green
basil, lemon	garlic*	poppy seed
bay leaves	ginger	rosemary
caraway	horseradish	saffron
cardamom	lemon balm	sage
cayenne*	lemongrass	savory, summer
celery seed	lemon verbena	savory, winter
chilli powder*	liquorice	sorrel
chives	lovage	tarragon
cinnamon	marjoram	thyme
clove	mustard seed	turmeric
coriander	nutmeg	vanilla – only the
cumin	oregano	real thing**
curry powder	paprika*	wasabi
		wild thyme

* Try to avoid strong flavours, such as chilli powder, cayenne, paprika and raw garlic, which may interfere with your hCG spray.
** If you do have to use vanilla extract or essence, please ensure that it is free from sugar, and preferably organic.

Stevia: sweet blessing

An exotic herb which grows in subtropical areas of South America, stevia is replete with non-caloric sugary molecules. This is the reason for its sweet flavour. Stevia has sweetened herbal drinks since pre-Columbian times. Its properties were first recorded in 1887 by a botanist named Antonio Bertoni, who wrote about the ways the natives of Paraguay used it. Others have discovered stevia in the past fifty years and made good use of it. Japan and the United States have done extensive research and safety-testing on the plant. Their research shows that this marvellous sweet herb is non-toxic, safe for diabetics and beneficial for weightloss, as well as for daily use for yourself and your family. More good news: stevia is not a source of nutrition for bacteria in the mouth, nor for yeasts and fungi such as *Candida albicans* in the body.

A few years ago, following some rather bogus animal research promoted by Monsanto – who produce many of the artificial sweeteners in the world – the European Parliament banned the sale of stevia in the UK and Europe. There is much pressure at the moment to lift that ban. In the meantime, if you live in the EU, you can, without difficulty, order stevia online from herbal shops, either in your own country or another European country, including the UK. It is widely available in shops and stores in the United States, Canada, Australia, New Zealand and most other countries of the world. Stevia is great for all sorts of reasons on Cura Romana.

How sweet is stevia extract?
Stevia extract is 200 times sweeter than sugar. Add a pinch to drinks like coffee or tea. Dilute in water when you are using it to make a salad dressing or dessert.

How many calories are in stevia extract?
None. Stevia extract has zero calories, zero carbohydrates, zero sugar, zero fat and zero cholesterol.

Can stevia extract replace sugar in the diet?
Yes. Refined sugar is virtually devoid of nutritional benefits and, at best, represents empty calories in your diet. Stevia is natural, much sweeter than sugar and has none of sugar's unhealthy drawbacks.

Can stevia replace artificial sweeteners in the diet?
Yes! Stevia is the only safe, calorie-free, all-natural alternative to artificial or chemical pharmaceutical sweeteners in the world.

Will stevia raise my blood-sugar levels?
Not at all. In fact, according to some research, it may actually lower blood-sugar levels.

Can I use stevia if I am diabetic?
Yes. Stevia is a great addition to a healthy diet for anyone with blood-sugar problems.

Vegetarian options

As you know, Simeons found it impossible to deal with vegetarians on Cura Romana. I, however, have worked with many vegetarians and find that they do well on the programme. In the process, I have developed some excellent protein alternatives. The principles of the Food Plan are the same for vegetarians as for the rest of us – four foods per meal and so forth. However, there are some great protein alternatives that even non-vegetarians tell me they enjoy while on hCG+Food Plan.

If, as a vegetarian, you can include fish and shellfish in your menus, this is ideal. It gives a lot of variety and fish is an excellent source of easily digested top-quality protein.

Here are some foods you can use as your protein source in place of meat or chicken:

1 White fish, from sole to cod to flounder, etc.

2 Prawns, shrimps, squid/calamari, lobster or crayfish.

3 An omelette made from one whole egg and three egg whites, cooked, of course, in a non-stick pan without oil.

4 100g of non-fat cottage cheese.

5 A smoothie made from 1 1/2 scoops of good-quality sugar-free micro-filtered whey. Vanilla works well. In the UK, Vital Whey is good. Solgar do a decent one which is available in many countries. Southern Hemisphere Red 8 is good – from the milk of New Zealand grass-fed animals. You can use your fruit allowances – strawberries, an orange, an apple – with some cinnamon or nutmeg if you wish. Best of all: make a green smoothie 'meal' containing 1 1/2 scoops of micro-filtered whey plus your allowance of raw green vegetables.

Go green for energy and health

To create a good alkaline balance, rejuvenate your body and regenerate your life, you need access to the *totality* of whatever greens you are using – don't just make your juice and toss the fibre away as most people do. Much like wholefoods, the best life-enhancing green liquids are those made not with a juice extractor but as 'whole juices', which means harvesting their goodness with the help of a powerful blender. This is something I value so much that I consistently travel with my Vita-Mix, the best in the world.

The fibre that is thrown away after ordinary juice extraction holds some of the most valuable treasures of the plant. Ordinary juicing produces only a fractured food, discarding much of the potent power the plant has to offer against ageing, illness and toxicity. It also wastes a lot of the plant's antioxidants. Get into whole juicing and you can toss out most of the expensive nutritional supplements you may have relied on to keep going. Whole green juicing does it better.

Your supermarket, your greengrocer and your garden offer a wide variety of organic green leaves ideal for whole juicing: kale, pak choi, mitsuna, lettuces, radicchio, spinach, turnip greens, grape leaves, Swiss chard/silver beet – the list is virtually endless. All these and more can be used to make a vegetarian meal on hCG+Food Plan or a meal replacement for non-vegetarians.

What is the secret of making green power drinks taste great? You can add your fruit allowance if you like, plus some stevia for sweetening, together with micro-filtered whey and your green vegetable allowance. This will create a total Food Plan lunch or dinner for you. Or you can choose, as I often do, to blend your green leaves with a little stevia and some chopped ice and have this together with a vegetarian omelette made with 1 whole egg and 3 egg whites. Then eat your allowed fruit on its own. Experiment to find out what works best for you. Blend and enjoy – not only while you are on hCG+Food Plan but on into Consolidation. I predict you will love green drinks so much that you'll continue to drink them long after your Cura Romana Journey is over.

So there we are. These are the basic things you need to know for your Cura Romana kitchen. Once you get the hang of preparing your hCG+Food Plan meals, it becomes a lot of fun. A great many people tell me when they have finished the hCG+Food Plan part of the programme, 'I'm really sorry it's over. I loved the simplicity of being able to eat that way. It was so satisfying and my foods have never tasted better.'

FOODS ALLOWED ON THE HCG+FOOD PLAN
(Days 3–24)

Breakfast	coffee (if you feel you absolutely must, but limit it to one cup a day)	Only 1 tablespoon of milk allowed each day. Use stevia for sweetening, as often as you like.
	tea – including herbal tea	As much as you like.

Lunch or dinner	meat – very lean and all visible fat removed:	100g of one lean meat or white fish, weighed raw and steamed, grilled or baked – no oil or fat is permitted.
	beef steak chicken breast (without skin) lamb goat hare rabbit veal venison other wild game	Avoid eating the same protein twice in one day. Go organic where possible!
	seafoods:	Sustainably sourced, preferably wild.
	bass clams cod crab crayfish flounder or other similar fish haddock halibut John Dory lobster mussels (green-lipped) oysters prawns scallops shrimps snapper sole squid/calamari tarakihi	
Vegetables	asparagus – 2 cups broccoli – 2 cups cabbage – 2 cups celery – 2 cups chicory – 2 cups cucumbers – 2 cups fennel – 1.5 cups	Only one kind of vegetable at each meal – no mixing. You can, however, always mix green leaves together in a salad and red cabbage with green cabbage in a salad.

	kale – 2 cups
	lettuce (any kind) –
	  2 cups
	onions – 1 cup
	red radishes – 1 cup
	rocket – 2 cups
	Swiss chard/silver
	  beet – 2 cups
	spinach – 2 cups
	tomatoes – 1 cup
		Avoid eating the same
		vegetable twice in one day.
		
		Limit your use of tomatoes to
		three meals a week. For
		some people they slow
		weightloss as they are very
		high in fruit sugar. Do not use
		cherry tomatoes – they are
		far too high in fruit sugar to
		use at all.
		
		Go organic where possible!

Fruit	1 medium apple
	
	1 small grapefruit
	  or 1/2 medium
	  grapefruit
	
	1 medium orange
	
	10 medium
	  strawberries
		Two fruits allowed per day.
		
		Avoid eating the same fruit
		twice in one day.
		
		Go organic where possible!

Breads, if desired	2 grissini/breadsticks	Not necessary, but fine if you want to eat them.

Seasonings	basil
	
	Bragg's Liquid
	  Aminos
	
	chives
	
	cumin
	
	fresh garlic – eat
	  only cooked garlic
	
	ginger, fresh root
	
	herbs, fresh organic
	
	lemon – juice only of
	  1 lemon (unless
	  otherwise specified)
	  each day
		Go organic where possible!

	Marigold Swiss Vegetable Bouillon or Rapunzel Organic Vegetable Bouillon	
	mint	
	mustard powder (incl Dijon) – calorie-free	
	parsley	
	pepper	
	salt	
	Tabasco	
	thyme	
	vanilla, the real thing	
	vinegar (incl apple cider vinegar	
	wasabi powder	
Milk	1 tablespoon	Only 1 tablespoon of milk allowed each day.
Drinks	coffee tea, including herbal tea water – fizzy, mineral or spring	**Note:** coffee can slow or stall weightloss in many people so restrict yourself to only 1 cup a day – if you feel you *must* drink it. If not, leave it out altogether. You can have these drinks (except coffee, which is dehydrating in nature) in any quantity and at all times of the day. You must drink between 2 and 3 litres of liquids a day.

Common Errors to Avoid on hCG+Food Plan

- Using contaminated spices – those filled with herbicides or pesticides, and/or irradiated. Also using spices that are past their sell-by date. Check carefully and buy organic. Many herbs and spices from supermarkets contain sugars (in various forms) or starches, and are often irradiated. Avoid them.
- Not drinking enough water. You need to drink 2.5–3 litres of water, herbal teas and other water-based drinks each day. Coffee doesn't count.
- Forgetting to take your fibre, vitamin C and senna tea.
- Eating fatty meat or exposing your hands, face or body to creams, fats and oils. Remember to remove all fat and skin from meat, chicken and fish before cooking. Use only mineral-based face and body products and never get conventional oils or creams on your hands. Wear gloves when preparing foods for others or washing greasy dishes.
- Not doing your two Feast Days properly when beginning the programme. They are important both for triggering weight-loss and for minimizing start-up hunger.
- Mixing vegetables at a meal. Simeons is clear about eating only a single vegetable at each meal. The only exception is leafy salad greens, which can be combined.
- Putting other things in your mouth, like gum. Even sugarless mints, gums, etc., interfere with the Protocol. Don't use them.
- Drinking diet drinks – including diet sodas. *Do not ever drink them. They cause weight gain and poison your body.*
- Weighing your 100g of protein *after* cooking. *Weight of protein you are eating has always to be its **pre-cooked** weight,* except when using tuna packed in water or brine.

- Eating the same protein, fruits or vegetables at both lunch and dinner. Your foods should be varied meal to meal.
- Eating too often in restaurants. Restaurants contaminate their foods with flavour-enhancers and other things that can interfere with your weightloss. If you must use a restaurant, order one steamed vegetable and plain meat, fish or chicken breast without skin – no fat. (Make sure you ask for your food to be weighed before it is cooked.) Or order an appetizer of tuna sashimi with an undressed green salad.

Plateaux – How to Handle Them

If your weightloss slows or stalls, don't panic. If you are cheating or being careless about measuring your foods: **STOP**.

Take a look at the list of most common errors above and consider some of the following fixes. Keep in mind that plateaux are not uncommon. Provided you are continuing to follow the Protocol precisely, weight stalls will pass. Some 'stalls' can be explained, such as when your weight arrives at old weight set points, or by the time of month, ovulation, steroids or sunburn. Other plateaux cannot be explained. What we are looking for is your overall average weightloss. It is completely normal for someone's weight to stall for a few days. *This does not mean you are not burning fat **provided you are following the Protocol exactly***. All plateaux will pass so long as you **stick to the Protocol**.

The following suggestions can help you both psychologically and physically to check out possible errors you may be making and to make it through any plateaux:

- Increase your water intake.
- Check on how your bowels are working. Are you using the tea or senna capsules, the fibre, the vitamin C every morning?
- Try adding a cup or two of white tea to your range of herbal teas.

- Don't eat the same fruit twice in one day. Or cut down on the size of the fruits you are using.
- Oranges, tomatoes and prawns stall some people. If you have been eating these foods, cut them down or out and see if weightloss speeds up. You may have a food sensitivity. To check this out, eat only one of these possible stalling foods at a time and only once every third day, then check out the speed at which you are shedding weight. If there is no difference, you can assume you have no problem with that food.
- Check your condiments for any form of sugar or suspected chemicals. 'Garlic salt' often contains sugar as an ingredient. Any seasoning salt or seasoning product must be carefully checked. In some countries this is impossible to do because ingredients are not listed on the package. Choose single organic herbs and spices to be safe.
- If you are mixing different kinds of vegetables at a meal, **STOP**.
- Try leaving out both *grissini*. You don't need them. You don't have to replace them with anything.
- Make sure there are no additives in chicken or other protein sources – often these are injected with some form of sugar, even in supermarkets.
- Check out the possibility that you might already be at your ideal weight. Are you hungry as well? First check that you are drinking enough water, then, if you are nearing the end of hCG+Food Plan, ask yourself if you are already nearing your body's ideal weight. If so, think about moving on to Consolidation.
- Is your period temporarily slowing things by encouraging your body to retain water?
- Have you changed or started one or more medications? Occasionally this can result in a few days' slowdown while the body adjusts.
- If you are experiencing a serious plateau – 4 days or more – do an Apple Day (see page 129). Simeons speaks of Apple

Days as being purely psychological in their effects, yet some people report a loss of 2 pounds the day after an Apple Day.

- Since the Protocol says you are not required to eat all the food each day, you may consider dropping one or both of the 'breads' and/or one of your fruits. Do eat your proteins and green vegetables, however, unless you are genuinely not hungry at one mealtime.
- Add a brisk walk to your day, a few minutes on a mini trampoline or some dancing. While vigorous exercise does not work for most people while on hCG+Food Plan, gentle exercise is great both for weightloss and for your mental, emotional and spiritual well-being.
- Make sure you get enough sleep.
- When you feel tired, rest. The programme brings some people so much energy that they forget to rest when their body is telling them to take a break. Take a nap, or spend some essential downtime listening to music or doing some quiet meditation. Listen to the natural rhythms and to the needs of your soul. Becoming aware of these energy shifts is a central part of the Cura Romana transformation. Now is the time to learn this art.
- Try adding a couple of tablespoons of organic apple cider vinegar to your daily regimen. You can use it on salads or steamed vegetables.

Weight stalls and Apple Days

Sooner or later – usually during the second half of a full course of hCG+Food Plan – your weightloss stalls for a few days, sometimes more than once.

Simeons, in his amazing intuitive genius – and I mean genius – devised something known as the Apple Day because he found that no amount of explaining to his patients why their weightloss was temporarily stalled, but would carry on again soon, satisfied them. (See explanation, page 85.)

If your weight does stall, of course you need to check to make sure that you're not suddenly putting your hands in oily water, or are not measuring your foods correctly (see possible errors, page 125). But if you are still continuing to follow the Protocol exactly, be reassured – your fat is still burning.

All that said, it can be fun to break through weight stalls by doing an Apple Day.

Apple Days

Here's how. An Apple Day starts at lunch one day and goes on until bedtime. What you do is take six beautiful large apples – the best that you can find – and you eat them whenever you like during the day. Six is the maximum you are allowed. If you only want to eat two or four, that's fine too. During the Apple Day, no other foods or liquids are allowed except for plain water. *You must only drink as much water as is absolutely necessary to wet your whistle – minute sips to quench your thirst if it becomes strong.* Most people find the apples keep them from being thirsty.

During your Apple Day you will still take your homeopathic hCG, but you will not take your fibre or your senna tea or capsules. The following morning, take your fibre and tea as usual and return to the normal diet Protocol.

How does an Apple Day work? Apples are a natural diuretic. Together with the fact that you are not having extra water on that day, they tend to draw the water out of the otherwise empty cells from which the fat has been burned. As a result, your weight shifts. Apple Days also spur the rapid elimination of waste, which can be good for improving the way that you feel in yourself. Often, when we are retaining water, we feel burdened. Apples are wonderful in other ways too. They are the richest fruit source of vitamin E and they offer a good supply of biotin and folic acid – which are two of the B-complex vitamins that are important in preserving energy and emotional balance. Apples are also a fine source of vitamin A and vitamin C – both natural antioxidants – as well as more than a dozen minerals, including sulphur, potassium, silicon, iodine, magnesium and calcium. And apples are also rich in a special form of soluble fibre called pectin which helps clear from the body heavy metals like lead and aluminium that we can pick up in our air, food and water.

An Apple Day is not something you need to use unless your weight has stalled for several days. And an Apple Day is not absolutely necessary, since plateaux get broken and the scales start showing weightloss sooner or later anyway. But, if you are feeling impatient, if you want to explore what an apple fast is like, or if you feel that it would benefit you to have a sense of breakthrough, then this is something that you might like to do. It is a fun experience which most people love. You can also read about Apple Days in Simeons' book.

Last-minute Notes

1 Tea, herbal tea, plain and sparkling water are the only drinks allowed. You can take them in any quantity at all times. Drink between 2 and 3 litres of these liquids a day. Many people are afraid to drink so much because they think it may make them retain more water. This is a wrong notion, as the body is more inclined to store water when your intake falls below its normal requirements.

2 Beware of coffee. It is best to leave it out altogether, but you can have one cup a day if you feel you must. In some people it slows weightloss. It can make you feel hungry. It also upsets blood sugar and slows down the process of connecting with your own innate energy source – an important and lasting experience on Cura Romana.

3 Go over every item on the list so that you are clear about what you are doing. No variations, other than those listed, may be introduced. Anything not listed is forbidden.

4 There is no objection to breaking up your two meals. For instance, you can have a breadstick and an apple for breakfast or an orange before going to bed, or a breadstick in the afternoon, provided they are deducted from your regular meals. You may not eat the whole daily ration of two breadsticks or two fruits at the same time, however; nor can you save any item from the previous day to eat the following day. You must also never eat more than the four items listed for lunch and dinner at the same meal.

5 Especially in the beginning, you will need to check and re-check every meal against your diet sheet before starting to eat. Never try to rely on memory.

Take your time

Go over again and again how the programme works and what foods you will and will not be eating. It is important that you, or whoever is preparing your food, understands how to carry out the food preparation with exactitude.

HCG+Food Plan Recipes

Most of the recipes you will find here are my own, developed out of my personal experience on the programme. A few of them have been given to me by men and women I have mentored. All are designed to provide you with a cost-effective collection to help you get the greatest enjoyment out of the simple, wholesome foods that are allowed on the Protocol. My intention in providing them is to inspire you to create your own recipes.

CHICKEN DISHES

One of the secrets for organizing yourself for hCG+Food Plan is to prepare in advance meals that you can take with you whenever neces-sary. Get to work ahead of time making a number of dishes you can refrigerate or freeze to use for several days. Or, when preparing dinner one night, double the amount of food you are preparing so that you have another meal for lunch or dinner the next day, or if you have to be away from home.

Chicken lends itself particularly well to this. The best way to prepare any chicken dish – which of course will always be a chicken breast without skin or fat – is to pound it with a meat tenderizer. What this does is break up the cross-links of protein, making it more tender and enabling it to absorb more flavours from any marinade or spices that you are using when you cook. This also prevents the chicken from becoming too dry and cardboard-like. It works the same way for meats, including game. When cooking chicken in a liquid, you can use 1/2 teaspoon of Marigold Swiss Vegetable Bouillon or Rapunzel Organic Vegetable Bouillon to flavour the liquid.

Steamed Chicken Breast with Basil

serves 1

A steamed chicken breast with cabbage, spinach, Swiss chard/silver beet or kale, this recipe is excellent cooked in an electric steamer.

WHAT YOU NEED

100g lean, skinless chicken breast with every bit of fat removed

2 teaspoons garlic, chopped

1 teaspoon dried basil or a handful fresh basil

2 cups raw red or white cabbage, spinach, Swiss chard/silver beet or kale, shredded

Himalayan or Malvern salt, to taste

HERE'S HOW

Cut the chicken into small cubes and place it in the little dish that sits inside the bottom of the steamer. Add garlic, basil and 1 tablespoon water. Place the vegetable in the top of the steamer and sprinkle with salt. Turn the steamer on for 20 minutes. As soon as the bell sounds, remove the vegetables from the top of the steamer, place them in a good-sized bowl and pour the chicken and juices from the dish over them. They bring wonderful flavour to the vegetables. Serve immediately.

> **Counts as one protein.**

Chicken Wrapped In Love

serves 1

If you love wraps and tacos, you will adore this one.

WHAT YOU NEED

100g lean, skinless chicken breast, finely chopped or ground just before cooking (you must do this yourself because if you buy ground chicken in a shop it will contain too much fat)

2 cloves garlic, chopped

1 tablespoon chopped yellow onion, onion granules or onion powder, to taste

1 teaspoon ground coriander or 1/4 teaspoon dried coriander

1/2 teaspoon Marigold Swiss Vegetable Bouillon or Rapunzel Organic Vegetable Bouillon powder

cajun seasoning (see page 163) or cayenne pepper, to taste

1 large green cabbage leaf

HERE'S HOW

'Fry' the chicken slowly, using only as much water as you need to do this. Add the garlic, onion, coriander and bouillon, plus more water if necessary. Simmer for a few minutes, being careful that you don't add either too much water, turning it into 'boiled chicken', or too little, making it dry out. While this is happening, lay your large cabbage leaf over the top of what you are cooking so that it softens and becomes malleable. When it is soft, remove it and put it on a plate. As soon as the chicken mixture is cooked, spoon it into the cabbage leaf and wrap the leaf around it.

> **Counts as one protein.**

Fiery Cajun Chicken

serves 1

This recipe includes Fiery Cajun Sauce (see page 156) as a marinade/cooking sauce. This dish is so fast and tastes so good that I make it frequently when I'm in one of my 'blonde' modes, in which I can't be bothered to spend the time thinking about what I want. You can also prepare it using a Sweet Wasabi Marinade or a Barbecue Sauce (see pages 159 and 161).

WHAT YOU NEED

100g whole lean, skinless chicken breast, pounded thin

1 serving Fiery Cajun Sauce

ground black pepper, to taste

HERE'S HOW

Lay the chicken breast in a grill pan, smother it in Fiery Cajun Sauce, sprinkle on pepper and grill each side until it's done.

> Counts as one protein.

Garlic Chicken Soup

serves 1

The fastest way of cooking chicken (or meat, for that matter) on Cura Romana is this little recipe. I made it up, fell in love with it and have used it again and again ever since. You can add a green vegetable, such as your daily allowance of chopped spinach, courgette or broccoli, or you can simply eat the chicken alone in the broth. I like to chop a lot of fresh garlic once a week, put it into a closed container and store it in the fridge so that I can go in and take out a spoonful whenever I want. As far as I'm concerned, the more garlic you put in this the better – but then I think I'm a garlic fanatic.

WHAT YOU NEED

100g lean, skinless chicken breast, cut into small cubes

1 teaspoon fresh chopped garlic

1 level teaspoon Marigold Swiss Vegetable Bouillon or Rapunzel
   Organic Vegetable Bouillon powder

2 teaspoons chopped parsley and/or 1/2 teaspoon lemongrass or
   1/2 teaspoon mild curry powder

180ml water

HERE'S HOW

Place all the ingredients in a saucepan and bring to the boil. Simmer
for 3–5 minutes and serve.

> Counts as one protein.

Zesty Lemon Chicken

serves 1

*So easy to make both for yourself and the family, all at the same time,
simply by increasing the amounts called for. You just have to make sure
that you are clear about how much belongs to you so that you stay
within the Protocol. This recipe works with fish and meat too.*

WHAT YOU NEED

white pulp scraped from 1/2 lemon

1 teaspoon Marigold Swiss Vegetable Bouillon or Rapunzel Organic
   Vegetable Bouillon powder

3 teaspoons Bragg's Liquid Aminos

dash of cayenne pepper

Himalayan or Malvern salt, to taste

pepper, to taste

60–120ml water

100g lean, skinless chicken breast, sliced thin and pounded (or use
   meat, game or fish)
zest of 1/2 lemon
juice of 1/2 lemon

HERE'S HOW
Add lemon pulp, bouillon powder, Bragg's and seasoning to water.
Simmer until all the liquid is soft and a little bit reduced. Add the
chicken or other protein and lemon zest and simmer just long enough
to cook it through. You may need to deglaze it every now and then by
adding more water if it gets too thick. Add the lemon juice and serve.

Counts as one protein plus half daily lemon allowance.

FISH DISHES

Fish is an excellent source of high-quality, low-fat protein. So are
shellfish – some of my favourite foods. If you love lobster, crayfish,
prawns, shrimps, crab, green-lipped mussels and scallops, this is a
great way to go for your proteins. Oily fish – such as salmon, mackerel
and sardines – are not allowed on hCG+Food Plan. Most white fish is
ideal.

There are many ways to cook seafoods. You can wrap them in
heavy foil or put them in a baking dish and bake them. You can steam
them in a steamer then cover them with a delicious sauce. I most often
simply squeeze part of my lemon allowance on to steamed fish and
serve.

When weighing shellfish, always remember to take them
out of their shells and make sure that they are at room temperature. If
you try to weigh shrimps, prawns or scallops frozen, their weights
will be distorted because, in their frozen state, they carry a lot of
ice.

Great Fish and Seafood Allowed on hCG+Food Plan

bass	John Dory	shrimps
clams	lobster	snapper
cod	mussels, green-	sole
crab	lipped	squid/calamari
crayfish	oysters	swordfish
haddock	prawns	tarakihi
halibut	scallops	tuna, fresh or
		tinned

Fabulous Fish Soup

serves 1

Fish soup is one of my favourite foods. I can never get enough of it. Here is one you can make and enjoy while on hCG+Food Plan.

WHAT YOU NEED

360ml water

1 teaspoon Marigold Swiss Vegetable Bouillon or Rapunzel Organic Vegetable Bouillon powder

1 teaspoon fresh chopped garlic, garlic granules or flakes

1/2 teaspoon onion granules or flakes

1 tablespoon fresh chopped basil leaves or 1/2 teaspoon dried basil

1 cup broccoli

100g white fish

1/4 teaspoon paprika or cajun seasoning (see page 163)

Himalayan or Malvern salt, to taste

pepper, to taste

HERE'S HOW

Put the bouillon powder, water, garlic, onion and basil in a saucepan and bring to a simmer. Add the broccoli and cook for 5 minutes with the lid on. Place the fish on top of the broccoli and sprinkle with paprika or cajun seasoning, salt and pepper. Put the lid on and cook for another 5 minutes.

> Counts as one protein plus one vegetable.

Yummy John Dory Bake

serves 1

Fast, delicious and good enough to serve to the whole family. This recipe takes only 15 minutes and is well worth the effort.

WHAT YOU NEED

100g John Dory or other white fish
juice of 1/2 lemon
1/2 teaspoon Himalayan or Malvern salt
1 teaspoon garlic granules, garlic powder or garlic flakes
1/2 teaspoon dried rosemary

HERE'S HOW

Place the fish in a ramekin. Pour the lemon juice over. Sprinkle on seasonings, cover with foil and bake at 175°C/350°F for 15 minutes until flaky. Serve immediately with a green salad.

> Counts as one protein plus half daily lemon allowance.

Fish Pesto

serves 1

This recipe calls for the juice of one lemon (all the lemon you are allowed in one day), so be careful not to use any lemon juice in any of your other meals.

WHAT YOU NEED

100g white fish

juice of 1 lemon

black pepper, to taste

1/2 teaspoon Marigold Swiss Vegetable Bouillon or Rapunzel Organic
  Vegetable Bouillon powder

2 cloves garlic, chopped

5–8 leaves fresh basil

3 tablespoons apple cider vinegar

Himalayan or Malvern salt, to taste

HERE'S HOW

Marinate the fish in lemon juice with black pepper for half an hour, then drain, saving the marinade. Slow-cook the fish in a shallow frying pan over a low heat for 2–3 minutes. While it's cooking, add the other ingredients to the marinade and purée them in a blender or food processor, adding a little bit of water if necessary for consistency. Pour the puréed sauce on to the fish and simmer for another 2–3 minutes over low heat.

Counts as one protein.

Prawns Marinara

serves 1

I have always loved marinara sauce – an Italian American sauce usually made with garlic, herbs, tomatoes and onions. This is my own hCG+Food Plan version. Traditionally, Italian Americans used it to add flavour to rice, pasta, seafood and pizzas. Now it is often used as a dipping sauce as well. It's great either way.

WHAT YOU NEED

1 cup chopped tomatoes (you can use a cup of tinned tomatoes if you wish, but in that case pour off some of the juice)
100g prawns, shells removed
1/2 teaspoon freshly grated ginger or 1/4 teaspoon dried ginger
pepper, to taste
1–2 cloves garlic, minced
5–6 chopped basil leaves or 1/2 teaspoon dried basil
1 teaspoon dried oregano
1/2 teaspoon chilli powder
Himalayan or Malvern salt, to taste

HERE'S HOW

Place half the diced tomato in a casserole dish. Sprinkle the prawns with ginger and pepper on both sides. Sear them for a moment on each side in a frying pan. Place the seared prawns on top of the tomatoes in the casserole dish. Add the minced garlic and the rest of the tomatoes, the basil leaves, oregano and chilli powder and place this mixture on top of the prawns. Season with salt. Cover the dish and bake at 175°C/350°F for 20 minutes.

> Counts as one protein plus one vegetable.

Sweet Lemon Fish

serves 1

This is a delicious dish that helps you use a rind from your daily lemon.

WHAT YOU NEED

1/2 lemon with rind

60ml water

1/2 teaspoon Marigold Swiss Vegetable Bouillon or Rapunzel Organic
   Vegetable Bouillon powder

1 tablespoon Bragg's Liquid Aminos

dash of cayenne pepper

stevia, to taste (optional)

100g white fish

1/2 teaspoon grated lemon zest

HERE'S HOW

Slice the 1/2 lemon into half again and add to the water in a pan. Boil
the lemon quarters until the pulp comes out of the rind. Add the
bouillon powder, Bragg's Aminos and cayenne pepper and stevia (if
using). Simmer over low heat for 5 minutes until the sauce has
reduced by half. Add the fish and cook for another 3–5 minutes,
deglazing periodically with water if need be. Garnish with the lemon
zest.

> **Counts as one protein plus half daily lemon allowance.**

Onion Caramelized Shellfish

serves 1

This dish works well with any kind of shellfish, as well as with all kinds of meat, chicken and game.

WHAT YOU NEED

60ml water

juice of 1 lemon

1/2 teaspoon Marigold Swiss Vegetable Bouillon or Rapunzel Organic Vegetable Bouillon powder

1/2 teaspoon organic vanilla essence (beware, it must be the *real* thing – no added sugar, preferably organic, not artificial 'vanilla flavouring')

stevia, to taste

Himalayan or Malvern salt, to taste

pepper, to taste

1 cup yellow onion, cut into rings

100g shellfish, fish or meat

HERE'S HOW

Heat the liquid ingredients except the vanilla essence in a frying pan with the bouillon. Add stevia, salt and pepper, onion and the protein food of your choice. Let it cook for another 2–4 minutes, then add the vanilla essence, deglazing with a little water as it's cooking to create a caramelized sauce.

> **Counts as one protein plus one vegetable.**

MEAT DISHES

By far the best meats are the wild meats, such as venison, wild goat, rabbit, hare, grass-fed beef or *extremely* lean lamb.

The leanest and healthiest beef comes from grass-fed animals. This means that the cattle are raised on grass from the time they are born until the day they are slaughtered. Sometimes, alas, even 'grass-fed animals' are stuffed on grains before they are slaughtered. This increases the fat content of the meat and also alters the kind of fat natural in animals fed on grass. So beware. The only acceptable lamb or beef on the programme is meat *at least* 93 per cent lean – in other words, which contains only 7 per cent fat or less. *Do not buy minced beef.* If you wish to use minced beef, mince it yourself at home. There is no way of guaranteeing the fat level in minced beef unless you know your butcher personally and make him understand that it must be this lean. The same is true of lamb. What I like to do is get my butcher to prepare for me 100g sirloin steaks, each of which is vacuum-packed separately. I get him to do the same with chicken breasts, in 100g portions and vacuum-packed, so that I can take a package out and cook it either from frozen or defrosted.

Here are a few of my suggestions for meat recipes. They apply equally to beef and all the other lean meats that are available to you.

Cook It Now – Eat It Later
serves 6

This is a convenient way of cooking chicken, venison, steak, prawns or other proteins so that you can then separate them into single-meal servings and take them with you wherever you go. I like to put single servings in a plastic bag and freeze them, then I can defrost them as I need them, eating them either hot or cold.

WHAT YOU NEED

600g pieces chicken breast, venison steak, prawns or other allowed
   protein

a marinade or seasoning of your choice (try Works-with-Everything
   Seasoning or Home-made Cajun Seasoning – see pages 162 and
   163).

HERE'S HOW

Either marinate the protein foods for half an hour, turning two or
three times, or press the spices into the surface of the protein foods.
Cook in a steamer or on a grill until done. Remove from the heat, cool,
then pack into separate packages and refrigerate or freeze for when
you need them.

It often works well to pound the uncooked proteins with a meat
tenderizer, but this is not absolutely necessary. It's just that they
absorb more of the marinades and spices if you do.

Counts as one protein.

Pan-seared Steak

serves 1

*This makes a delicious gourmet main meal that is quick and easy to
prepare. It can be adapted to different kinds of meat, from beef and
venison to wild goat, lean lamb and veal. Though Simeons did not use a
wide variety of meats – most were not available in Italy at the time he
wrote – all these meats work very well on Cura Romana. They are lean,
they have no extra fat on them and are much lower in calories
than domestically farmed animals. Try them and I think you'll be
delighted.*

WHAT YOU NEED

1 rounded teaspoon chopped fresh garlic

1/2 teaspoon freshly ground black pepper

1/2 teaspoon flaky sea salt

1 teaspoon ground cumin

1/4 teaspoon cayenne pepper

100g medallion lean beef, veal, venison or wild goat

HERE'S HOW

Gently blend the spices together then pour them on to a flat plate. Roll and pat the medallion into the spices until all sides are coated. Put the meat in a heavy pre-heated pan or under a grill and cook for 2–3 minutes a side (depending upon whether you want your meat well done or rare).

One medallion serves one person. It can be useful to cook four or five at a time. Once they are cooked you can freeze them in separate bags and thaw them whenever you need them. They are great to carry with you when you are out during the day or in the office working.

> **Counts as one protein.**

Easy Chilli

serves 1

This is a delicious dish which you can serve on top of steamed greens, broccoli or other permitted vegetables. It's quick and easy to make, especially if you cook the meat first.

WHAT YOU NEED

100g game (venison, rabbit, hare, wild goat – one of my participants from Norway even prepared it using reindeer; you can fall back on ultra-lean beef if nothing else is available)

1 cup diced tomatoes

1/2 teaspoon Marigold Swiss Vegetable Bouillon or Rapunzel Organic Vegetable Bouillon powder

dash of cayenne seasoning or chilli seasoning

2 teaspoons finely chopped garlic

1/2 teaspoon cumin

1/2 teaspoon onion granules or flakes

1/2 teaspoon freshly grated ginger root or 1/4 teaspoon dried ginger

240ml water

HERE'S HOW

Make sure you mince your meat by hand or dice it very finely yourself. Dry-fry it until almost cooked, then add the rest of the ingredients and simmer until done.

> **Counts as one protein plus one vegetable.**

Beef Bourguignon

serves 1

WHAT YOU NEED

100g ultra-lean beef, cubed

1 tablespoon chopped raw onion

1 tablespoon chopped raw garlic

240ml hot water

1 teaspoon Marigold Swiss Vegetable Bouillon or Rapunzel Organic
   Vegetable Bouillon powder

1 whole tomato, chopped

1/4 teaspoon cumin

pinch of marjoram

Himalayan or Malvern salt, to taste

pepper, to taste

HERE'S HOW

Braise the cubes of beef together with the onion and garlic, add the
other ingredients and slow-cook for half an hour until the beef is
tender. Add extra liquid as necessary to get the right consistency.

Counts as one protein plus one vegetable.

Spaghetti
serves 1

This is a fun recipe if you are a spaghetti-lover. It's made from whatever kind of ultra-lean meat you choose, chopped fine or minced – it must be 93 per cent lean. The spaghetti is replaced by shredded white cabbage.

WHAT YOU NEED

100g 93 per cent lean minced meat

2 cloves garlic, chopped fine

1 onion, cut into small pieces

2–3 teaspoons fresh basil or 1 teaspoon dried basil

1/4– 1/2 teaspoon home-made cajun seasoning (see page 163)

1/4 teaspoon dried oregano

Himalayan or Malvern salt, to taste

pepper, to taste

1/2 cup tomatoes

2 cups finely shredded white cabbage

HERE'S HOW

Dry-fry the minced meat with the garlic, onion and seasonings, adding salt and pepper to taste. Add the chopped tomato and simmer over low heat for 10 minutes. Serve over steamed, finely shredded cabbage.

Counts as one protein plus one vegetable.

SALADS AND VEGETABLES

The best way to eat any of your vegetables on hCG+Food Plan and ever afterwards is raw. Cucumbers, onions and asparagus are all delicious raw. So are all the green vegetables that we use to make salads. You can dress vegetable dishes with one of the sauces and dressings (see pages 155–64) or, if you prefer, simply shake on some apple cider vinegar, fresh garlic, salt and pepper with a dash of Bragg's. Then you needn't bother to make a dressing. Apple cider vinegar is good to use on Cura Romana as it encourages fat-burning.

You will remember that Simeons specifically insisted that you eat only one of the allowable vegetables at a meal. I, however, find that in many cases – once you have finished the first week to ten days of the programme and provided your weightloss is going well – you may get away with mixing your vegetables. *What you do not want to do is eat too many tomatoes, because they are very high in fruit sugar. As far as cherry tomatoes are concerned, don't touch them* – they are even higher in fruit sugar. Eating some grated onion on top of a spinach salad or making a salad from shredded cabbage to which your allowable fruit – say an apple or an orange – is added can make a delicious salad.

There are two great ways to make salads while on hCG+Food Plan. You can either make a salad as a side dish entirely on its own, put together from a single vegetable, or – if you find that mixing vegetables does not interfere with weightloss – you can combine all sorts of wonderful things, like cucumber and orange, for instance, or fennel and asparagus. The other way is to use your vegetables as a base for other foods, making, for instance, a spicy crab salad, a lobster salad, a crayfish salad, a chicken salad and so forth. Either way works beautifully and gives you a great deal of variety. Here are a few suggestions to get you started.

Orange and Fennel Salad

serves 1

This is a delicious and uplifting combination that works beautifully with whatever you are preparing as your protein foods.

WHAT YOU NEED
juice of 1/2 lemon
fresh mint or coriander, chopped
stevia (optional)
1 orange, pips removed, cut into segments
1 raw fennel bulb, grated

HERE'S HOW
Combine all the ingredients in a bowl and chill. Top with Roman Orange Vinaigrette (page 159) and serve.

> Counts as one vegetable plus one fruit plus half daily lemon allowance.

Apple Slaw

serves 1

Sweet and lovely.

WHAT YOU NEED
2 cups finely shredded white or red cabbage
1 apple, diced
1/2 teaspoon chopped fresh garlic
dash of ground cinnamon
Himalayan or Malvern salt, to taste
pepper, to taste
stevia, to taste

HERE'S HOW

Put the cabbage in a bowl and add the apple and garlic. Sprinkle with cinnamon and season with salt and pepper. Dress with Vinaigrette Dressing (page 162), add stevia and serve.

Counts as one vegetable plus one fruit.

Japanese Cucumbers
serves 1

I learned this recipe from the Japanese family with whom I grew up. I have slightly modified it for hCG+Food Plan.

WHAT YOU NEED

2 cups thinly sliced cucumber

2 tablespoons apple cider vinegar

1 tablespoon Bragg's Liquid Aminos

1 teaspoon finely grated red onion

pinch of ground coriander

cajun seasoning (see page 163) or cayenne pepper, to taste

HERE'S HOW

Mix all ingredients together and leave to marinate for 15 minutes. Serve chilled.

Counts as one vegetable.

Curried Chicken Salad

serves 1

This is a good whole meal in itself.

WHAT YOU NEED

1 teaspoon chopped fresh garlic

curry powder, to taste

stevia, to taste (optional)

2 tablespoons Bragg's Liquid Aminos

juice of 1/2 lemon or 1 tablespoon apple cider vinegar

2 cups diced celery

100g steamed chicken breast, cut into small cubes

HERE'S HOW

Mix the garlic and curry powder with the liquids and pour over the celery to cover completely. Leave to marinate for 15 minutes. Add the cubes of chicken, either hot or cold, and serve immediately.

> Counts as one protein plus one vegetable.

Spicy Prawn and Mesclun Salad

serves 1

WHAT YOU NEED

100g cooked prawns, weighed without shells

Sweet Wasabi Marinade (page 159)

pinch of tarragon

Himalayan or Malvern salt, to taste

pepper, to taste

1 cup chopped celery

1 cup mesclun salad

Mix the prawns with the marinade, tarragon and seasoning. Serve over chopped celery and mesclun.

> Counts as one protein plus one vegetable.

Steamed Coriander Cabbage
serves 1

Quick and easy, you can make this recipe in an electric steamer while you are cooking your protein food. I like to chop the protein foods into small pieces and serve on the cabbage. You can substitute Swiss chard/silver beet or spinach for the cabbage.

WHAT YOU NEED
2 cups cabbage or Swiss chard/silver beet, shredded
several sprigs fresh coriander or 1/2 teaspoon ground coriander
juice of 1/2 lemon
zest of 1/2 lemon
2 teaspoons calorie-free mustard
Himalayan or Malvern salt, to taste
pepper, to taste

HERE'S HOW
Place the greens in the steamer and steam for 5–10 minutes until tender. Meanwhile, mix together the coriander, lemon juice, lemon zest and mustard. Put your steamed vegetables in a bowl, add the lemon juice mixture and toss. Sprinkle with salt and pepper. Serve immediately.

> Counts as one vegetable plus one half daily lemon allowance.

SAUCES, SOUPS AND DRESSINGS

Trusty Teriyaki Sauce
serves 1–2

This is great as a liquid in which to cook fish, chicken or meat. It can be used either as a marinade or as a cooked sauce. The more you simmer it, the more intense its flavours become.

WHAT YOU NEED

120ml water

1 teaspoon Marigold Swiss Vegetable Bouillon or Rapunzel Organic Vegetable Bouillon powder

2 tablespoons apple cider vinegar

juice of 1/2 lemon

pulp and juice of 1 orange

1/2 teaspoon freshly grated ginger (you can use ground ginger if you must)

1/2 teaspoon finely chopped garlic (more if you like)

zest of 1/2 lemon

zest of 1/2 orange

stevia, to taste

HERE'S HOW

Put all the ingredients in a small saucepan and bring to a simmer. Continue to simmer for 15–20 minutes until the liquid is reduced. As it simmers, add a little water or broth to intensify the flavours.

> Counts as one fruit.

Fiery Cajun Sauce

serves 1

This is great as a dressing for salads or as a dipping sauce for fresh vegetables. It also makes a good marinade for fish, chicken or vegetables.

WHAT YOU NEED

3 tablespoons apple cider vinegar

juice of 1/2 lemon

1/4– 1/2 teaspoon cajun seasoning (see page 163)

stevia, to taste

1/2 teaspoon chopped fresh garlic or garlic flakes

1/2 teaspoon chopped onion or onion flakes

1/2 teaspoon freshly grated ginger or a generous pinch of ground
   ginger

HERE'S HOW

Put all the ingredients into a small blender and mix well. Serve.

Counts as half daily lemon allowance.

Bragg's Liquid Aminos and Mustard Marinade

serves 1

I created this recipe one day when in a hurry to grill a small steak on my George Foreman grill. I was longing for something that had a little bit more spice to it and I didn't have time to create a proper marinade or let the meat sit in it for long. It works equally well with fish and chicken. It calls for Bragg's and Home-made Mustard (page 164) or mustard powder.

WHAT YOU NEED

3 tablespoons Bragg's Liquid Aminos
2 teaspoons calorie-free, organic Dijon mustard or 1 teaspoon
   mustard powder
freshly ground black pepper

HERE'S HOW

Put all the ingredients in a shallow bowl or dish. Mix together quickly. Add your meat, chicken or fish to the marinade and turn over a couple of times while the grill is heating (you can also make this in a pan if you prefer). Place the protein on the grill or in the pan and pour the rest of the marinade over the top. (If using a George Foreman grill, be sure you collect all the juices as they run off into the collection pan.) Cook rapidly – it takes about 3–4 minutes. Remove from the grill or pan and pour the extra liquid over the protein. Serve immediately.

> Marinade itself counts as zero calories.

Salsa

serves 1–2

Salsa is something you can always fall back on to spice up your meals. It makes a wonderful sauce for a Cura Romana omelette (which you make with 1 whole egg and 3 egg whites). It is also delicious on fish, chicken and minced meat.

WHAT YOU NEED

1 cup fresh chopped tomatoes

juice of 1 lemon

3 cloves garlic, minced

2 tablespoons finely chopped onion

1 teaspoon fresh oregano or 1/4 teaspoon dried oregano

1 tablespoon fresh chopped coriander or 1/4 teaspoon ground coriander

1 tablespoon apple cider vinegar (optional)

dash or two of green Tabasco sauce

Himalayan or Malvern salt, to taste

freshly ground pepper, to taste

HERE'S HOW

You can purée the ingredients in a blender or food processor if you like, but I prefer them chunkier, so I tend to chop them, adding all the spices at the same time. If possible, refrigerate for at least half an hour – even better, overnight – to allow the flavours to develop.

Counts as one vegetable plus one daily lemon allowance.

Sweet Wasabi Marinade

serves 1

Wasabi is something I absolutely adore, not only spread on fish but on steaks – occasionally even on chicken.

WHAT YOU NEED

3 tablespoons Bragg's Liquid Aminos

juice of 1/2 lemon

1/4–1/2 teaspoon wasabi powder, depending on how brave you are (I always seem to overdo it)

stevia, to taste (if you want it sweet – I often make it sour)

HERE'S HOW

Mix the liquids together, then blend in the wasabi powder, taste and add stevia if you like.

> Counts as half daily lemon allowance.

Roman Orange Vinaigrette

serves 1

This is easy to prepare and goes well with rocket, spinach or any fresh green-leaf salad. It also makes a delicious marinade for fish and chicken.

WHAT YOU NEED

1 orange

1 tablespoon apple cider vinegar

juice of 1 lemon

2 small cloves garlic, chopped, or a generous pinch of garlic flakes

pinch of Himalayan or Malvern salt

dash of green Tabasco sauce or cayenne (optional)

freshly ground black pepper

stevia, to taste

HERE'S HOW

Combine all the ingredients in a blender and blend until smooth. Pour over your salad. Garnish with 1 teaspoon orange zest and more freshly ground black pepper.

> Counts as one fruit plus one daily lemon allowance.

Tomato Basil Vinaigrette
makes 2 servings

Good for dressing any kind of fresh salad.

WHAT YOU NEED

2 tablespoons tomato paste
juice of 1/2 lemon
3 tablespoons apple cider vinegar
60ml broth (made with 1/2 teaspoon Marigold Swiss Vegetable
   Bouillon or Rapunzel Organic Vegetable Bouillon powder) or water
1 teaspoon finely chopped onion or onion flakes or powder
1 teaspoon finely chopped fresh garlic
chopped fresh basil leaves, to taste, or 1/2 teaspoon dried basil
pinch of oregano
dash of green Tabasco sauce or cayenne pepper
stevia, to taste

HERE'S HOW

Mix all the ingredients together in a blender. You might prefer them heated, in which case you can bring the mixture to a boil and simmer for a few minutes. I prefer the ingredients raw. Chill and serve over salad with freshly ground black pepper.

> Counts as half daily vegetable allowance.

Barbecue Sauce

serves 1

This is a great sauce to use on chicken, fish, meat or even an omelette (provided you do not have any trouble with tomatoes, as a few people find that eating them slows down their weightloss – keep an eye on this).

WHAT YOU NEED

1 cup chopped tomatoes, fresh or tinned (pour off the liquid if using tinned – use only the tomatoes)

juice of 1 lemon

1 tablespoon finely chopped onion

2–3 cloves chopped fresh garlic

1 teaspoon chopped fresh herbs – parsley, chives, coriander, basil, etc.

cayenne pepper or cajun seasoning (see page 163), to taste

1/4 teaspoon Marigold Swiss Vegetable Bouillon or Rapunzel Organic Vegetable Bouillon powder

few drops hickory-flavoured liquid smoke (optional)

1/4 teaspoon celery seeds

60ml apple cider vinegar

Himalayan or Malvern salt, to taste

pepper, to taste

stevia, to taste (if you like the traditional sweet barbecue-sauce flavour)

HERE'S HOW

Place all the ingredients in a food processor and blend. Pour into a saucepan and bring to the boil. Simmer for 5–10 minutes. Add more water if necessary to keep the sauce from drying out. Smear over cooked meat, chicken, fish or an omelette. Cook and serve.

> Counts as one vegetable plus one daily lemon allowance.

Vinaigrette Dressing
serves 3–4

WHAT YOU NEED

6oml apple cider vinegar

6oml water

1/2 teaspoon chopped fresh garlic

good pinch of cajun seasoning (see page 163)

good pinch of onion salt

1/2 teaspoon zero-calorie mustard

Himalayan or Malvern salt, to taste

pepper, to taste

stevia, to taste

HERE'S HOW

Mix all the ingredients in a jar and shake well, or blend in a blender. Store in the fridge and use as needed.

Works-with-Everything Seasoning

This is a seasoning I use all the time. It works beautifully on salads, protein dishes and in soups. Keep it in an airtight container.

WHAT YOU NEED

1/2 teaspoon garlic flakes

2 teaspoons ground coriander

2 teaspoons ground cumin

1 teaspoon Himalayan or Malvern salt

a pinch of chilli powder

1 teaspoon black pepper

1/2 teaspoon mustard powder

HERE'S HOW

Mix all the ingredients together thoroughly (I use a mortar and pestle). Store in an airtight container away from heat and light.

Home-made Cajun Seasoning
makes enough for several meals

This is a gourmet's delight. You can make it with either fresh or dried herbs. In either case, always refrigerate it. Fresh herbs will last for 2 weeks in the fridge, the dried herbs for several weeks.

WHAT YOU NEED

1 teaspoon paprika

1/2 teaspoon freshly ground pepper

1/2 teaspoon ground cumin

1/2 teaspoon mustard powder

1/2 teaspoon cayenne pepper

2 teaspoons fresh thyme or 1/2 teaspoon dried thyme

1 teaspoon Himalayan or Malvern salt

2 teaspoons fresh oregano or 1 teaspoon dried oregano

2–3 garlic cloves, well mashed, or 1/2 teaspoon garlic flakes

3 dessertspoons grated onion or 1/2 teaspoon dried onion flakes

HERE'S HOW

Combine all the ingredients by hand. Store in an airtight jar. Use immediately or store in the refrigerator.

Home-made Mustard
makes enough for several meals

A great no-calorie mustard which you can make and keep in the fridge for up to 2 weeks.

WHAT YOU NEED

2 tablespoons mustard powder

1 tablespoon finely chopped fresh garlic or 2 teaspoons garlic flakes

3 teaspoons onion flakes

1/2 teaspoon freshly grated ginger or 1/4 teaspoon ground ginger

1/2 teaspoon grated horseradish (optional)

120ml apple cider vinegar

3 tablespoons water

pinch of cayenne pepper

Himalayan or Malvern salt, to taste

pepper, to taste

stevia, to taste

HERE'S HOW

Mix all the ingredients together and heat in a saucepan for 2–3 minutes, adding a little extra water if you need it.

SWEET TREATS

Strawberry Sorbet
serves 1

This recipe is equally delicious made with strawberries, oranges or grapefruit.

WHAT YOU NEED
a handful of frozen strawberries, a frozen orange with peel removed
   or a frozen grapefruit with peel removed
3 large ice cubes
stevia, to taste
1/2 teaspoon pure vanilla essence (the *real* thing, no sugar – go
   organic)
3 tablespoons water

HERE'S HOW
Place all the ingredients in a blender and blend until smooth, but do
not let it become completely liquidized. Serve immediately.

> Counts as one fruit allowance.

Hot Spiced Orange

serves 1

Back in the 1950s hot spiced orange tea was a Christmas favourite along with mulled wine. It must be served hot to work, and be sure to use the cloves. Without them this luscious drink loses its kick.

WHAT YOU NEED
pinch of ground nutmeg
pinch of ground cloves
pinch of ground cinnamon
1/4 teaspoon pure vanilla extract (the *real* thing, preferably organic)
stevia, to taste
1 orange, sliced thinly crosswise
zest of 1/4 of the orange

HERE'S HOW
Combine the spices with the vanilla extract and stevia. Add the sliced oranges and the zest and heat gently, adding a small amount of water as necessary. Cook for 2–3 minutes. Serve hot.

Counts as one fruit.

Frozen Grapefruit Rounds

serves 1

This makes a surprisingly delicious frozen treat or dessert.

WHAT YOU NEED
1/2 grapefruit, peeled and sliced in thin rounds
juice of 1/2 lemon
1/4 teaspoon grated lemon zest
stevia, to taste (this works best with Spoonable Stevia by Stevita, but you can also use the powdered white stevia if you prefer)

HERE'S HOW

Dip the grapefruit rounds in the lemon juice, then coat with lemon zest and stevia. Freeze until hard.

Counts as one fruit plus half daily lemon allowance.

Vanilla Apples
serves 1

A wonderful apple dessert that you can make for the whole family if you like. It leaves everyone with a warm feeling.

WHAT YOU NEED

juice of 1/2 lemon

1 tablespoon apple cider vinegar

1/4 teaspoon pure vanilla essence (the *real* thing, no sugar, preferably organic)

stevia, to taste

1 apple, peeled, cored and thinly sliced

a very small pinch cinnamon

HERE'S HOW

Mix the lemon juice, vinegar, vanilla and stevia in a small saucepan. Add apple slices and heat gently. Serve warm, sprinkled with cinnamon.

Counts as one fruit plus half daily lemon allowance.

DRINKS

Extract of Ginger Tea
serves 1

One of my favourite drinks on Cura Romana is made from tincture of ginger. You can buy it in any shop that sells pure herbal tinctures and it isn't expensive if you buy 100 or 200ml. You use very little each time and it makes a wonderful, warming drink. It helps counteract fatigue, improves digestion and it is just all-over delicious. Alternatively, you can use fresh ginger, as detailed below.

WHAT YOU NEED
1/4–1/2 teaspoon freshly grated ginger, to taste
1/4–1/2 teaspoon stevia (optional)

HERE'S HOW
Pour boiling water over the freshly grated ginger, add stevia and drink immediately.

Vanilla Tea
serves 1

This is a delicious treat, wonderful when you feel that you need something sweet to indulge yourself.

WHAT YOU NEED
1 teaspoon pure vanilla extract (the *real* thing – no sugar, preferably organic)
1/4–1/2 teaspoon stevia (the best is Spoonable Stevia by Stevita but any will do)

HERE'S HOW

Pour boiling water over the vanilla extract and stevia and serve immediately. It's also a great 'dessert' after any meal.

Orange Frappe
serves 1

This is my version of a drink that was invented accidentally by a restaurateur at a trade show in Greece. You must use sparkling water for it to bring the 'kick' that is its signature.

WHAT YOU NEED

1 orange, peeled and pips removed

3 ice cubes

stevia, to taste

1/4 teaspoon pure vanilla essence (the *real* thing – no sugar, preferably organic)

sparkling water – enough to fill a large glass

HERE'S HOW

Blend the orange, ice, stevia and vanilla essence. Add sparkling water and serve.

Counts as one fruit.

HCG+FOOD PLAN – QUICK GUIDE

QUESTIONS, QUESTIONS

Q: I want to do Cura Romana but my significant other disapproves. What can I do?

A: Give him or her this book to read. It is easy for someone who knows nothing about the Protocol to be worried about you embarking on it. Show your partner the research. This can help him or her understand the nature of the programme, how it has been used successfully by hundreds of thousands of people, how health-enhancing it can be. Tell him or her that you want his or her love and support. Ultimately you are the one responsible for what you choose to do for your health. Honour that.

Q: Will I experience hunger while I'm on the Protocol?

A: It would be natural for you to feel a little hungry before lunch and dinner, although some people report days when they do not even experience this. Everyone is different. About 60 per cent of people report little or no significant hunger right from the very first day. Others report feeling low to moderate levels of hunger off and on for the first few days as the homeopathic and Food Plan bring about shifts in the way their body is functioning. It is extremely rare for anyone to experience strong hunger during the Protocol. I have not encountered this in any of the people I have personally mentored.

Q: If hCG brings about weightloss, why don't pregnant women lose weight?

A: Many actually do. In men and non-pregnant women, hCG works to turn the body's inessential fat stores into energy only when there is a significant decrease in calories and fat. This is why the homeopathic hCG works only when used in conjunction with Simeons' exacting Food Plan. It is not the hCG itself that brings about your weightloss, but the combination of the homeopathic with this very specific low-calorie diet that turns your body's inessential fat stores into usable energy.

Q: Will my metabolism slow down on Cura Romana?

A: No, it will not. Cura Romana is not like ordinary weightloss diets, which compromise muscle and bone and cause metabolism to slow down. It draws energy from and burns up only your inessential fat stores, and this it does only in combination with a very specific low-calorie diet. In this case, in effect, the hCG triggers the body to turn stored fat into vitality, decreasing excess fat reserves but not compromising muscle, so there is no resulting slowing of metabolism.

Q: Won't I lose the same amount of weight just eating a very low-calorie diet without the homeopathic hCG?

A: Good question. You might well lose the same amount of weight eating fewer calories, but you would need phenomenal willpower and you would lose weight not only from your *inessential* fat stores but also from your *essential* fat stores. This is what makes people look so haggard and feel so weak on conventional weightloss diets, as often both muscle and bone are lost before inessential fat. This is also what causes metabolism to slow down, and makes them highly prone to regaining weight easily and laying down more abnormal fat in the process. Conventional dieting also brings about a loss of bone density. Homeopathic hCG together with Simeons' Food Plan mobilizes only the abnormal fat in the body, turning it into energy and preventing the immediate refilling of emptied fat cells. This is how it helps you shed excess fat without undermining bone, muscle or metabolism.

Q: Should I worry if I am light-headed, or weak or tired?

A: This experience is not uncommon for some people – especially those who begin their programme with what I call a *fatigue deficit*, often from weeks or years of driving themselves too hard or from a lot of unwise yo-yo dieting in the past. This has no effect on the speed or effectiveness of weightloss. It is, however, a call to rest. Do it. I have experienced this myself. I took naps on many days at the beginning of the programme and then on the odd day when the fatigue returned afterwards. Take an Epsom salts bath (see pages 94–5). Give yourself time to write in your journal about whatever comes up without censoring anything you put down – positive or negative. Use a good B12 Energy Booster spray – 3 sprays under your tongue and hold it there for 30 seconds – twice a day. Rest, even if only for 5 minutes at a time. As the fatigue deficit clears, your energy should build steadily.

Q: Can I drink coffee?

A: Simeons allowed his patients to drink as much coffee as they wanted. But that was more than fifty years ago, before insulin resistance, leptin resistance and food intolerance burgeoned to epidemic proportions as a result of all the grain-based carbs, sugars, junk fats and convenience foods on which our society feeds. I strongly advise anyone going on Cura Romana to stop drinking coffee altogether *before* beginning the Protocol. At the very least, I suggest you limit yourself to one cup a day. There are several reasons for this:

1 Coffee can slow or halt weightloss in 80 per cent of people on the programme because of the way it triggers blood sugar and insulin release.

2 It depletes B vitamins important for good brain and nervous-system functioning.

3 It undermines adrenal functioning and can lead to adrenal exhaustion.

4 Coffee does not provide you with energy. What it's providing is chemical stimulation and the perceived 'energy' comes from your body's struggle to adapt to increased blood levels of stress hormones. In most cases this induced emergency state leads to well-defined side-effects. Collectively they are known as 'caffeinism'. Ironically, caffeinism is characterized most strongly by fatigue.

Most important of all: one of the greatest gifts of Cura Romana is your coming to discover your own natural source of energy and vitality from within. Drinking coffee on the programme only defers your being able to do this. Please remember: everything you need is *inside you.* You need to tap into your own font of endless vitality and live from that.

Q: What if I have a detox reaction?

A: A headache, a rash, itchy skin, if they occur, are most likely to be signs of wastes being released from your system. This can happen very rapidly on the Protocol – especially at the beginning. Take an aspirin and get some rest if you have a headache. It will pass in a few hours; in *rare* cases, when the body is quite toxic before beginning the programme, it may take a few days. Use calamine lotion on a rash. Take an Epsom salts bath. Get some extra rest. Ask your body how you can help it. I am quite serious about this. Listen gently and it will tell you.

Q: *What can I do for dry skin?*

A: Use QV Lotion or liquid paraffin. Get yourself some plain aloe vera gel (make sure there are no oils mixed with it – you want the kind that can be taken orally), then put it in a spray bottle and spritz your skin with it. Use petroleum jelly for dry lips. Order some TwinLab Na-PCA Non-Oily spray online. Be patient. My own legs felt like alligator skin for the first week or so whilst on the Protocol. That is how I discovered the wonders of QV Lotion. I ordered some and by the time it arrived my skin had become as smooth as a child's thanks to the alterations in hormonal balance that hCG+Food Plan had brought about in my body.

Q: *I lost 8 pounds in the first week but now I'm losing only half a pound a day and some days nothing at all. What am I doing wrong?*

A: Nothing – provided, of course, that you have been following the Protocol to the letter. Do check back and read about common errors to make sure. Changes in the speed of weightloss and weight stalls are completely normal. As Simeons says, 'There may be no drop at all for two or three days and then a sudden loss which establishes the normal average. These fluctuations are entirely due to variations in the retention and elimination of water, which are more marked in women than in men. A plateau always corrects itself, but many patients who have become accustomed to a regular daily loss get unnecessarily worried and begin to fret.' If the stall lasts for more than three days, do an Apple Day (see page 129).

Q: *Are there other bonuses from using hCG and Simeons' exacting food Protocol?*

A: Yes. People often feel terrific during and after the programme. Once they are into hCG+Food Plan and then Consolidation, they don't experience the irritability or weakness common to weightloss diets. They look years younger. The majority of people sleep better, yet many people find that they need to sleep less. They experience a continual slimming in the shape of the body. They report how wonderfully their clothes fit as the body remodels itself and restores its natural contours. All such experiences are unique to Cura Romana.

Q: What if I get a cold or flu while I'm doing Cura Romana?

A: The good news is that these minor ailments tend to be less virulent while on hCG+Food Plan – easier to manage and over more quickly. This may be because one of the bonuses of hCG during pregnancy is the natural immune-system enhancement it brings to the body. My way of dealing with these infections is to increase the frequency of the 3,000mg of vitamin C you are taking as part of the programme from once a day to three or four times a day until two days after all symptoms have cleared. Most important: get some extra rest and take Epsom salts baths.

Q: Do I have to eat the full 500 calories each and every day?

A: Simeons says, 'Those not uncommon patients who feel that even so little food is too much for them, can omit anything they wish.' That being said, it is my experience that it is important for everyone to eat their protein foods and green vegetables twice a day. Weightloss is better when you do. You can certainly eliminate the *grissini* and the fruit with no problem. And, if you are genuinely not hungry and are feeling well, you can certainly skip the odd meal if you like. What you must not ever do is stop eating for a couple of days or more in the belief that this will help you lose weight faster. It won't. It could make you unwell.

Q: Are there clinical complications from using Cura Romana?

A: Not when it is used correctly. Even the injections of hCG that

Simeons used were minute doses – 125 IU per day – compared to as much as one million IU of hCG per day excreted in the urine of pregnant women. As far as the homeopathic form of hCG is concerned, there have been no complications reported by anyone so far. Again, it is important to reiterate that the Cura Romana Protocol which uses hCG in its homeopathic form plus Simeons' very specific dietary regime is *essential* for successful weightloss on the programme. Too many healthcare professionals and amateurs have sought, and continue to seek, to change or 'improve' Simeons' method, sometimes out of ignorance and at other times because of a desire to sell a lot of unnecessary products to people for financial gain. It is essential that the programme be honoured in all its elegance. *Exactitude, guidance and careful monitoring of what you are eating while on the Protocol are essential for your success.*

Q: How safe is homeopathic hCG?

A: The homeopathic hCG used in Cura Romana is a safe and very stable compound homeopathic remedy. Several potencies are used together, some of which contain none of the original substance – only its molecular energy blueprint. People who have used both the homeopathic and the injectable report that there is no difference between them in terms of the effectiveness and speed of weightloss they bring. The advantages of homeopathic hCG are many. They include not having to have injections and being able to carry your hCG around with you so that you can use it three times a day, even if you are out and about. Perhaps the most interesting and valuable advantage of all is that, when properly formulated, the homeopathic form of hCG brings a tremendous sense of lightness and transformation to people mentally, emotionally and spiritually. It not only reshapes their bodies but many claim it reshapes their whole lives. Again and again we hear that they have never felt as well physically or as good about themselves as after Cura Romana.

HCG is one of the very few drugs of totally natural origin that remain part of the medical pharmacopeia. Because of its ability to simulate ovulation, hCG has been used for a very long time in fertility treatments. It is also used in the treatment of boys whose testicles have not descended. All hCG is manufactured in laboratories after extracting natural hCG from the urine of pregnant women. It is interesting that, since 1930, no complications have ever been reported in relation to its manufacture.

Q: Should I tell my doctor what I am doing?

A: If you are on any prescription medication, it is important that you let your doctor know that you intend to carry out the Cura Romana programme and, if he asks, suggest he reads this book. Also, give him a link so he can download Simeons' book from *www.curaromana.com*. Your doctor will need to check whether the dosage of any medication you are on needs to be adjusted as you undergo your Cura Romana Journey. So improved are most participants' health parameters that doctors frequently need to reduce the dosage of any medication they are prescribing for them. In some cases your health improves so much that you end up no longer needing medication, even if you have been taking it for a long time.

If, on the other hand, you suffer from gout, gallstones, diabetes or have recently been treated for a coronary occlusion, it is important your doctor monitors your progress while you are on the programme. These conditions are not contra-indications for Cura Romana, but in such cases, as Simeons says, the Protocol needs to be carried out under the watchful eye of a wise physician.

Q: Will I be hungry during the hCG+Food Plan?

A: You'll feel little or no hunger on the programme because the hCG is mobilizing fat efficiently. This naturally decreases the appetite, so even though you are taking in fewer calories, your body is able to access energy stored in your fat cells. A very small number do feel hungry occasionally. This can be a sign of low blood sugar or a consequence of an overgrowth of fungus or yeast in the body, which often clears in the process. People report that they feel a little bit hungry before lunch and dinner, which is normal and what we want. About 60 per cent of people say from the very first day they experience no hunger. Sometimes it takes between two and five days for hCG+Food Plan to kick in so that unnatural hunger disappears. Once the body becomes familiar with the hCG+Food Plan process, most people have masses of energy and feel terrific on the programme.

Q: How much weight can I expect to lose on Cura Romana?

A: This varies from person to person. Women usually lose between 15 and 20 pounds a month, while men can shed between 20 and 30 pounds. A few people lose 10–12 pounds in the first week. On average, women lose from 0.5–0.6 pounds a day. One of the remarkable things about the programme is that, even when weightloss slows down temporarily, you continue to lose inches, so that after a certain length of time you experience either a large drop in the scales and/or your clothes literally seem to be falling off.

Q: Is Cura Romana some kind of magic wand?

A: No, it is not. Cura Romana can do its work only if you are willing to work with it by making sure that you follow the Protocol exactly, both during the hCG+Food Plan rapid weightloss period and during Consolidation. It is the partnership that is formed between you and the programme that makes permanent weightloss happen.

Q: Will I lose muscle mass on Cura Romana?

A: No. Cura Romana is unique among weightloss programmes. It only targets inessential fat stores and it spares muscle tissue. This is why your skin grows firmer on the programme, your natural body shape emerges and you can continue to build strength throughout the nine-week Cura Romana Journey.

Q: Do I need to exercise?

A: No. Weightloss on Cura Romana does not depend on exercise. It takes place because of shifts in metabolic functions whether or not you exercise.

Q: What about wrinkles and stretch marks?

A: On Cura Romana abnormal fat deposits diminish. Troublesome fat from double chins, pot bellies and thick thighs is often the first to go. The programme does not deplete structural and essential tissue necessary to maintain healthy body function, as do ordinary weightloss diets. The body rejuvenates itself both inside and out, giving people on the programme a fresh, glowing appearance. Unlike conventional slimming diets, it does not result in wrinkles and stretch marks. Rather, skin seems to become more toned through the process.

Q: Can I go on taking my nutritional supplements?

A: On hCG+Food Plan you must not take any supplements except vitamin C. The oil-based vitamins, including supplements such as CoEnzyme Q10, omega-3s, vitamins E and A, will interfere with weightloss. Simeons wrote that every time you lose a pound of fatty tissue, only the fat is burned up. All the vitamins, all the protein, the blood and the minerals that this tissue contains in abundance are fed back into the body. Simeons wrote, 'We have never encountered a significant protein deficiency nor signs of lack of vitamins in patients.' As soon as you get into Consolidation, you can go back to taking your supplements as before.

Q: Does Cura Romana have other benefits?

A: It does. It appears to regenerate the body's essential fat tissues – the structural fat around organs and fat deposits – and other fat stores which are essential for health but which never distort the shape of the body and which help protect us in times of famine. This makes your skin, face, neck and hands look renewed and glowing. Most conventional weightloss diets take away structural fat as well as inessential fat. It is this which creates the sunken, hollow appearance and the deep fatigue common with yo-yo dieters. On hCG people report having more energy, a decreased appetite and fewer food cravings than ever before. Homeopathic hCG and the exacting Food Plan bring natural appetite control. It also helps prevent new fat from filling in the empty spaces after excess weight is lost.

Q: Can I continue to take my medications?

A: Yes. It is important that you consult with your doctor or healthcare practitioner before discontinuing any medication. That being said, if you are on medication for diabetes, depression, cholesterol, high blood pressure, etc., it is essential that your healthcare professional monitors the changes in the medical parameters on which the dosages of your drugs have been based. The improvements in these areas that take place on Cura Romana can happen rapidly and your doctor will want to decrease the amounts he is prescribing for you. You do not want to be on a high level of medication to control blood pressure when your natural blood pressure has already dropped significantly. This can occur within the first two weeks on hCG+Food Plan. Blood pressure tends to normalize, as do cholesterol readings; arthritis symptoms lessen or disappear and so forth. It is important that your healthcare practitioner knows this and takes whatever action is appropriate.

Q: Do I have to be very fat for the programme to work or can I do it just to help reshape my body?

A: This is an effective Protocol for anyone who carries abnormal fat deposits. Even if you need to shed only 10 or 15 pounds, you can use it to reshape your body and enhance your health.

Q: Do I need to eat grissini – the breadsticks?

A: No. If you know your body does not handle wheat or other cereals and grains well, you should avoid them altogether. You do not have to replace them with anything – just leave them out. For people who respond poorly to starchy foods or gluten, they can trigger cravings and slow weightloss.

Q: I get cramps in my legs at night – what should I do?

A: Cramps are caused by a deficiency in magnesium or potassium. It happens to perhaps two people out of 100. Take 300mg of magnesium in the morning and evening along with approximately 100mg of potassium.

Q: How long will it take before I begin to see and feel results?

A: By the end of the first week on Cura Romana your body can begin to reveal a new sleek, toned appearance and feel. By then, you are also likely to sense a new balance in your emotions and the beginnings of a new outlook on your body and your life.

Q: Can my teenage son or daughter do the programme?

A: Yes. Provided they have completed puberty – from sixteen onwards – and are genuinely motivated to do so. You must never try to press the programme on anyone who is not absolutely committed to doing it. That would be an infringement of their personal freedom to choose. It would also lead to failure.

Q: Does Cura Romana work for men?

A: Yes, it does. It's used with equally good results in men and women. Homeopathic hCG has no negative effects on male hormones. In fact, it works even better and faster for men than it does for women.

Doctors actually prescribe injectable hCG to enhance natural testosterone production while preventing testicular atrophy during a course of male hormone replacement therapy. It is even given to men whose natural testosterone production has been undermined as a result of over-use or abuse of steroids. I had one man on the programme who was very heavy and, within the first three weeks, shed more than 40 pounds. The average weightloss for a man is a pound or more a day.

Q: What should I say to people who ask what I am doing?

A: It's often best to say nothing. If you tell them you are on a 'diet' they are going to ask things like 'What do you eat for breakfast?' or, since they are uninformed about the unique nature of the Protocol, make comments like, 'Only five hundred calories a day? That's dangerous.' Wait until you are well into the programme and your body and face are so transformed that people start to remark on it. Then you can refer them to the book if they are genuinely interested. Otherwise thank them and reply, 'Yes, I've been feeling very well lately.'

PART THREE

THE

CONSOLIDATION

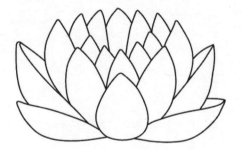

Now or For Ever
– You Choose

S IMEONS GAVE FAR too little advice on how to follow Consolidation in order to maintain weightloss permanently. Because of this he was only able to report 60–70 per cent success with his Cura Romana patients.

> **Simeons says:** *When the three days of dieting after the last injection are over, the patients are told that they may now eat anything they please, except sugar and starch, provided they faithfully observe one simple rule. This rule is that they must have their own portable bathroom-scales always at hand, particularly while travelling. They must without fail weigh themselves every morning as they get out of bed, having first emptied their bladder. As a general rule one can say that 60%–70% of our cases experience little or no difficulty in holding their weight permanently.*

So far our Cura Romana Consolidation programme has enabled 95 per cent of the men and women who have followed it to make weightloss last. It is not based on following by rote what you can and can't eat the way you had to while you were on hCG+Food Plan. It has been designed to enable you to discover the foods that your unique body *loves* and therefore thrives on, as well as those foods your body *hates* – foods that destabilize energy and emotional balance, and undermine the proper functioning of the hypothalamus and your autonomic nervous system, causing your body to retain water and gain weight. Although there are some basic guidelines on protecting your body from weight gain, the foods that you identify will be individual to you. Once you discover them, you will find that your body can eat as many as it likes of the former group provided you cut out the latter. It is as simple yet as life-changing as that.

Right now, as far as weight is concerned, your aim should be to help your body become familiar and comfortable with your new set point – the weight you are now – so that it can remain at this weight. To do this, you will need to follow Consolidation with the same precision, awareness and accuracy you used while on hCG+Food Plan. Keep reminding yourself: the goal of Consolidation is to help your metabolic reset become permanent.

A Backward Glance

Let's go back and review how this metabolic reset has taken place. Remember, hCG is a complex protein-based hormone with receptor sites in the diencephalon area of the brain. Your homeopathic made use of the body's hormonal signalling pathway to alter the functioning of the diencephalon, bringing about rapid weightloss, altering hunger perception and rebalancing hormones. It took some time for the homeopathic to make good connections with these receptors and teach the cells new ways of functioning. Consolidation's goal is to make sure this reset lasts.

Beware Over-enthusiasm

Consolidation is *not* a time for you to try to lose more weight. If you still have more weight to lose, that's fine. After Consolidation has finished you can do another spate of hCG+Food Plan followed by another Consolidation.

> **Simeons says:** *The . . . trouble which is frequently encountered immediately after treatment is again due to over-enthusiasm. Some patients cannot believe that they can eat fairly normally without regaining weight . . . They try more or less to continue the 500-calorie diet on which they felt so well during treatment and make only minor variations, such as replacing the meat with an egg, cheese, or a glass of milk. To their horror they find that in spite of this bravura, their weight goes up. So, following instructions, they skip one meagre lunch and at night eat only a little salad and drink a pot of unsweetened tea, becoming increasingly hungry and weak. The next morning they find that they have increased yet another pound. They feel terrible, and even the dreaded swelling of their ankles is back.*

During the three weeks you spent on hCG+Food Plan, you were eating minimal protein. Protein is a key component of Consolidation. It is imperative that, during these six weeks, you build up your protein stores. If you intend doing another Cura Romana Journey after Consolidation, the proteins and green vegetables you eat during this time are also crucial to prepare you for a second Journey during which you will shed yet more of your inessential fat.

Protein has unique metabolic characteristics which are central to Cura Romana. Do not skimp on it as you begin Consolidation. Listen to your body and allow it to eat all it wants. Protein foods require energy to burn – what is known in medical terms as *postprandial thermogenesis*. When you are eating good-quality foods – that is, good-quality organic meat of all kinds, fish, eggs and top-quality micro-filtered whey – you can actually increase the caloric needs of your body's metabolism thanks to the added energy used in digesting these foods. As you enter this six-week period, be sure to concentrate on two categories of food: green vegetables and top-quality – presumably, therefore, animal-based – proteins.

> **Simeons says:** *During treatment the patient has been only just above the verge of protein deficiency and has had the advantage of protein being fed back into his system from the breakdown of fatty tissue. Once the treatment is over there is no more hCG in the body and this process no longer takes place. Unless an adequate amount of protein is eaten as soon as the treatment is over, protein deficiency is bound to develop, and this inevitably causes the marked retention of water known as hunger-edema.*

What was happening to those of Simeons' patients who, out of fear of regaining their weight, limited the foods they were eating in an attempt either to prolong weightloss or prevent weight gain after hCG+Food Plan, is this. Their food choices, combined with anxiety and a mistaken understanding of what was expected of them, had led to their having destabilized the metabolic reset. Simeons knew that the way to correct this was by feeding them protein. Why? Because protein foods remind the diencephalon that it is to continue to function in the way it has learned to function while on hCG+Food Plan. This knowledge formed the basis of his correction for their problems.

> **Simeons says:** *The treatment is very simple. The patient is told to eat two eggs for breakfast and a huge steak for lunch and dinner followed by a large helping of cheese and to phone through the weight the next morning. When these instructions are followed a stunned voice is heard to report that two pounds have vanished overnight, that the ankles*

are normal but that sleep was disturbed, owing to an extraordinary need to pass large quantities of water. The patient, having learned this lesson, usually has no further trouble.

Simeons' intuitive awareness of the power of top-quality protein foods also led him to create his 'Steak Day' as a rapid correction on Consolidation. You will learn about this later (see page 225–6).

Welcome Back to Old Favourites

As soon as Consolidation begins you can go back to using whatever creams, lotions and oil-based make-up you like. You can also ease yourself back into exercise if you wish. But please do not do this because you believe you should, or out of fear that if you don't exercise you won't maintain your weight. Choose the kind of exercise you like best, whatever that happens to be. You can have massages again now too, using oils if you like. You can even enjoy a glass of good wine with a meal during Consolidation – provided of course that you find out first that your body wants a glass of wine. Some bodies don't, believe it or not. A number of men and women I have mentored who were inveterate wine-drinkers before Cura Romana have found – usually to their surprise – that they no longer enjoy it.

Finally, you can return to taking nutritional supplements if you like. Before Cura Romana you may have taken a lot of vitamins and minerals, green supplements and the like. You might be surprised to find how few you seem to need now that your body has become so much better balanced. I personally take little more than a good food-state vitamin and some omega-3 oils. (Be sure to check periodically on *www.curaromana.com* for updates on the best vitamin and mineral supplements and how to order them.)

Food-State Vitamins

Food-state vitamin manufacturers grow the majority of the foods and botanicals that go into their formulas. Then, using state-of-the-art scientific instrumentation, they test, validate and document the potencies of all the raw materials that make up the formula. This is achieved by using high-performance liquid chromatography to test vitamin potency and inductively coupled plasma optimal-emission spectrometers to test mineral potency. They are also very careful in how they handle the food extracts that are often added to these supplements. For instance, they use a very specific system of drying which transfers heat gently and efficiently, removing moisture from delicate foods and botanicals while preventing oxidation of the raw materials. This protects the integrity of the food and the botanicals as well as protecting against the degradation of their nutrient content, maintaining the colour and the flavour.

Because the natural food-state vitamins are indeed natural and food-state, you will find that the recommended daily serving of vitamins per person is usually somewhere between six and eight tablets a day in order to be able to obtain the full benefit. In addition to the usual vitamins, i.e. vitamin A, C, D3, E, K1, folate, and so forth, there should be a good broad spectrum of minerals: calcium, iodine, magnesium, selenium, chromium, molybdenum, manganese, etc. These wonderful food-state vitamins also often contain extracts taken from other plants that are beneficial to the body – things like extract of barley grass and green papaya, extract of carrot, for instance, as well as astragalus and many of the Ayurvedic herbs or the herbs that are used in Chinese medicine – reishi and shiitake mushrooms, foti and kudzu root. This is the kind of vitamin that I think you will benefit most from.

The problem is that most vitamins sold in stores and online are synthetic man-made vitamins that have been produced in the laboratory in an attempt to match the molecular structure of naturally occurring vitamins normally found in our foods.

Unfortunately, our bodies have been accustomed to absorbing with ease the vitamins and minerals that we get from our foods and these man-made synthetics, even though they try to match the molecular structures, are not the same – our body does not handle them as well. So you may be taking a high-potency vitamin that has come recommended and you may not actually be absorbing the vitamins and minerals it contains. This is one of the reasons why I am so passionate about whole-food, natural multi-vitamins and minerals.

Consciousness Holds the Key

Becoming aware of your body as your best friend, nurturing it, honouring it and loving it as it is right now can make Consolidation a life-changing passage. It's exciting to discover the foods that work for you and those that don't. Eliminating from your life those that don't helps maintain a high level of wellness, makes you resistant to infections and early ageing, while keeping you lean and strong as the years pass.

Again and again, after completing nine weeks on Cura Romana, people tell me, 'It feels to me that I've been this weight *always*. I can hardly remember that once I was so much heavier or that I once fought food cravings and felt desperate about my body.' In Consolidation you learn systematically about establishing new eating behaviours. They develop naturally to support your body and your sense of self-worth permanently. Before long, the emotional and spiritual expansion that so often accompanies Cura Romana becomes just a way of life.

Simeons never allowed his patients to count calories. Nor do I. Counting calories creates a feeling of having to 'control' everything. This is not what re-educating appetite and establishing a new set point is about. That being said, neither is Consolidation a time for gleefully mixing together different foods. Your body has become beautifully clean and balanced. Make use of this. You now have an unparalleled opportunity to test out your foods and find out what works for you. So, during the first week, go easy. Don't flood your system with too much food all at once. Increase the quantity and variety of foods step by step. Don't confuse your system by eating, say, grapes and nuts and cheese all at the same time. You have been living on small quantities of high-quality, simple foods – proteins, non-starchy vegetables and two servings of low to medium glycemic fruit. Stick as much as possible to the same *kinds* of foods and let your natural appetite determine how much you want of each.

Some Cura Romana participants assume that, having been through hCG+Food Plan – a powerful tool for rapid, healthy weightloss – they will now be able to eat whatever they like and automatically maintain the new weight. This is not the case.

The Way Ahead

If you want to make your weightloss last – along with all the bonuses that have come with it – you will learn in the next five chapters how you can make it happen. To make Consolidation with all its own bonuses work for you, you will need to do three things:

1 Listen to your body in order to respect your own essential being.

---

2 Work with both in a practical way, identifying the foods your body loves and those it hates.

3 Honour both by eating as much as your body wants of the foods it loves while eliminating those it hates.

Just as hCG+Food Plan is a simple but profound process, so is Consolidation – but in a whole new way which brings new gifts in its wake. Carried out with awareness, the next six weeks help you discover a new, sensuous and fun relationship with food.

Decisions, Decisions

Let's get back to that decision. You are free to choose to do this or not. You can go back to old habits, allowing your weight gradually (or not so gradually, should you choose to make fish and chips, pizza and doughnuts your daily fare) creep up. After all, you will have learned by now that hCG+Food Plan works for safe, simple, rapid weightloss. You can always tell yourself that you can go back next year and do it again. The only negative involved, if you choose to go down this route, is that the health and emotional benefits you have gained in the past few weeks are likely to become things of the past instead of the future as the metabolic reset destabilizes as a result of feeding your body on foods it is unable to handle well.

If you choose not to follow Consolidation as it is written – and it took me almost three years to work this out so that it really is effective – you will not only undermine your ability to make your weightloss last and be free of all those cravings you used to have – far more importantly, you will undermine the diencephalic reset that has brought you greater emotional balance, a better ability to deal with stressors in your life, and all the other health benefits from the programme. These, by the way, are not mere consequences of weight being lost but, at a fundamental level, are the result of the better functioning of your entire autonomic nervous system, at the core of which lie the hypothalamus, thalamus and pituitary in the diencephalon.

It's time for you to decide which way you want to go: permanent or temporary? What matters most is that you take responsibility one way or the other. Remind yourself that you are not a victim of circumstances beyond your control as you might once have believed. You are free to follow whichever path you choose. Get clear about what you want. Then make your decision and follow it.

The Low-down

L ET'S CUT TO THE CHASE.
The culprits that made you gain weight were not fats or lack of exercise but the carbohydrates you ate – specifically the cereals, grains, starches and sugars.

As soon as you eat these foods, three significant things occur:

● They are quickly turned into glucose, flooding your blood-stream with sugar.
● They induce food cravings and addictive eating.
● They trigger insulin release from the pancreas.

Sound Nutrition

If you love researching things in depth, do read *Good Calories, Bad Calories* by Gary Taubes (see page 206). The information and research it contains are the best I have ever found. There is also a wonderful practical book, *Nourishing Traditions* by Sally Fallon, Mary R. Enig and

Pat Connolly. It not only offers a wealth of unbiased nutritional information about fats, proteins and enzymes but also includes lots of delicious recipes. It could be called the bible of good nutrition and good eating and is based on the work of Weston Price, who wrote the classic *Nutrition and Physical Degeneration* after travelling the world and studying the consequences of introducing Western food practices to indigenous cultures back in the 1930s and 1940s. However, when using any cookbook, no matter how good, it is important to remember that your body and your metabolism are unique to you. Just because there is a lovely recipe for wholemeal bread does not mean that this is something that you should be eating. (See page 348 for further information on this book.)

Fast Track to Fat

If you are someone with a diencephalic imbalance or a genetic tendency to gain weight, eating these carbohydrate foods will make you fat. They will also encourage the development of any number of chronic conditions, from aches and pains, sleep troubles and hormonal imbalances to depression, addictions and early ageing. They will also prevent you from making your weightloss permanent. Even in people who do not have an inherited tendency to gain weight, a diet high in cereals, grains and sugars is a major contributor to coronary heart disease, cancer, Type 2 diabetes and virtually all the degenerative conditions known as the diseases of civilization.

From a scientific point of view, carbohydrates are nothing more than organic compounds made of carbon, hydrogen and oxygen. Ideally – that is, in the body of someone who is young and healthy with no inherited tendency to weight gain – grains, cereals and sugars are meant to be turned into glucose to supply fuel for most of the body's organs. But throughout the history of human civilization – ever since the agricultural revolution – these foods have been manipulated, used and abused in any number of ways, all of which point down a road that ends in premature ageing, physical degeneration and obesity.

Simple and Complex

Nutritionists divide carbohydrates into two categories – simple and complex. All carbohydrates are made up of simple sugars called mono-saccharides: such as fructose, glucose and galactose. These monosaccharides link together into twos called disaccharides and then form longer chains called polysaccharides or starches.

Simple carbohydrates are often referred to as 'refined' carbohy-drates. These include sugar, honey and other obviously sweet foods, as well as breads, flours, cereals and white rice. These are digested and assimilated quickly – leading to a rapid rise in blood sugar and insulin secretion. For years we've been told to eschew *simple carbs* in favour of *complex carbs*.

Some examples of complex-carb foods include wholemeal bread, brown rice, wholemeal pasta, potatoes, dry beans, carrots and corn. All grains are starchy carbohydrates. However, whole grains – such as wholewheat pasta – are considered better for you because they also have more fibre, contain more vitamins and minerals and, of course – most important – are unrefined. Although they too turn into glucose, they do this more slowly than do the simple carbs. Having said this, however, it is important that you know that the number of overweight people who do not even handle the so-called 'good complex carbs' is legion. It is your job, while on Consolidation, to discover how your own body responds to them.

Complex carbohydrates are made up of more complicated chains of sugars and contain more fibre than their simple cousins. Because your body assimilates them more slowly, complex carbs cause a more moderate insulin and glucose response, provided you do not eat too many of them.

But here lies the rub. Even complex carbohydrates can be prob-lematic for people who have a tendency to gain weight. Just like simple carbs, they end up as glucose in your bloodstream. When you eat more than your metabolism can efficiently turn into energy, the glucose from them is converted into fat in your liver or shunted directly into the fat cells, causing weight gain. This is especially true of someone who has insulin resistance and in whom the hypothalamic function has become distorted as a result of having consumed a diet high in sugar and grain-based carbs over a long period of time.

Knock, Knock – No Answer

Glucose is burned in your cells to produce energy. It is derived from the foods you eat and makes its way into the bloodstream where it is ready to be taken up by your cells and used. It can get into your cells, however, only in the presence of the hormone insulin. Your pancreas releases insulin into the bloodstream so that it is able to bind with receptor sites on your cells – in much the same way that a key fits into a lock. The door that insulin unlocks is the one through which glucose passes into cells. Without insulin, the glucose from your food knocks at the door. No matter how hard it tries to get into your cells where it can be turned into energy, there is no answer. For when chronic high levels of insulin are present in the blood, the cell receptors stop responding to it and glucose can't find a way in to be turned into ATP – your body's energy currency. This is called insulin resistance – the major instigator of obesity.

From an evolutionary point of view, the hormone insulin evolved as the body's prime mechanism for storing excess carbohydrate calories in the form of fat in order to protect us from famine when it occurs. This is why insulin promotes the accumulation of body fat in a highly aggressive way – especially in those of us who gain weight easily.

Good Carbs, Bad Carbs

When you eat low-starch vegetables such as broccoli, spinach, asparagus and cauliflower, or proteins such as fish, meat and eggs, the levels of glucose in the blood rise very slowly and modestly. On the other hand, when you eat what are known as high-glycemic foods – those foods that produce high levels of blood sugar almost instantaneously, like a muffin, pasta, breakfast cereal or ice cream – your blood sugar soars. Then the pancreas shunts more insulin into your bloodstream. Large doses of circulating insulin send the message to your body to 'store fat'.

Once this vicious scenario begins, your body is in trouble. You gain more fat. This increases insulin resistance yet more and releases free fatty acids into the blood, which in turn further increases insulin resistance. You end up with adipose deposits which distort your body and which, even if you starve yourself, seem impossible to shift.

This phenomenon is what Simeons likened to the 'deposit account' of fat from which you cannot draw energy. Increased insulin levels have sent messages to the body to store grains, cereals and sugars in the form of fat and have instructed it not to let go of that fat. The grains and sugars you eat not only make you fat, they make sure that you stay that way. For instead of burning fat as fuel, the insulin response has to be moderated. This is exactly what Cura Romana does, amongst many other things, and the only way to protect the metabolic reset it brings about is by avoiding grains, starches and sweets.

You know that feeling you can get when you still feel hungry although you've just eaten a meal? Following a meal or snack containing grains, cereals and sugar, blood sugar rises, insulin is secreted in order to control it and very quickly this causes hunger. This is a major reason why cravings and food addictions are such a common experience amongst people who are overweight and whose metabolism has therefore become distorted. What happens? You reach for more grain-based carbs and sweets. If you don't eat you can feel ravenous, shaky, moody, depleted. For many overweight people this creates a chronic situation in which you never get rid of the stored fat and you are continually dealing with a rollercoaster of energy dives.

Addictive eating

All starchy vegetables, sugars and grains are *addictive*. The fewer you eat of foods from this category, the more easily will you maintain your normal weight permanently. Conventional slimming diets do not work because, unlike Cura Romana's ability to bring about a diencephalic reset, they provide no way of breaking the vicious cycle of insulin rise, fat storage and cravings. Blood sugar and insulin levels remain high, further decreasing the body's ability to burn fat and creating addictive eating, much of which is often blamed on emotional issues when in fact it is a highly biochemical phenomenon.

Age Fast

Insulin resistance and high levels of circulating insulin in the blood do something else directly related to fat distortions in the body. When insulin levels are high, they suppress glucagon and human growth hormone. Glucagon is a hormone that encourages the burning of fat and sugar. Growth hormone is essential for the health of muscle tissue and for building new muscle mass. In effect, the combination of insulin's action on glucagon and human growth hormone not only feeds obesity, but makes your body fat and flabby.

A diet high in cereals, grains and sugars (which happens to be the way of eating for 90 per cent of the Western world) is the fastest way to speed the ageing process because the tissues in your body become progressively more tolerant to high levels of insulin. Eventually you develop insulin resistance syndrome (Syndrome X). Excess insulin is also behind the development of serious degenerative conditions. It:

- stimulates cancer-cell growth
- causes Type 2 diabetes
- raises cholesterol
- shortens lifespan
- creates auto-immune diseases
- increases addictions and food cravings
- increases blood pressure
- triggers irritable bowel syndrome

In light of all this, let's revisit for a moment prehistoric eating habits. The carbohydrates our Palaeolithic ancestors ate came not from grains, cereals and sugars but from wild herbs and vegetables gathered by foraging. Although these plants are also 'carbohydrates', they bear little resemblance to the highly cultivated fruits and starchy vegetables that we eat today. Our ancestor's vegetables were more like kale and Swiss chard/silver beet, a leafy green vegetable similar to spinach which very few people eat now. They ate little fruit. In the northern latitudes fruit was seldom eaten at all except for small, wild fruits which looked more like rose hips than the fruits on our supermarket shelves. The plants our ancestors ate had much more fibre than modern plants do. As a result, Palaeolithic humans got about five times more fibre than we do.

There is a lot to be said for vegetable-based fibre. First, foods high in vegetable-based fibre take time to eat and require a lot of chewing. This in itself gives a sense of satisfaction and fulness. Plant-based fibre slows the digestion of any plant starches and buffers any natural sugars that they contain. In this way, fibre-rich plant foods minimize sharp rises in glucose and insulin. Virtually all the Palaeolithic plant foods were fibre-rich. Our early ancestors rarely ate grains or cereals, which in any case had to be gathered from wild grasses and other plants that bore no resemblance to today's top-heavy, carb-rich, cultivated varieties. The problem with modern foods is that most are manufactured from grains in a highly refined form. They are shunted from the bloodstream very quickly and can, as we have seen, wreak havoc with our insulin and blood-sugar levels, producing peaks and troughs of energy, cravings, chronic fatigue, insulin problems and weight gain.

For Ever Lean

Now that the appetite- and weight-control mechanisms in the brain have been reset on hCG+Food Plan, what are the most important things for you to remember if you never want to gain weight again? Here they are:

1 Obesity is a disorder of fat accumulation. It is not caused by over-eating. Nor is it caused by lack of exercise.

2 Insulin is the primary regulator of fat storage. Whenever insulin levels are high, either long-term or simply after eating a meal, fat accumulates in our tissue. When insulin levels are low, our body is able to release fat from fat deposits and turn it into energy – provided, of course, that the hypothalamus in the diencephalon area of the brain is functioning properly.

3 The *natural fats* you eat, whether saturated or unsaturated, are not the cause of heart disease, obesity or other chronic diseases of civilization, despite what we've been taught.

4 Grain-based and cereal-based carbohydrates are the major culprit behind weight gain and one's inability to shed fat. They negatively affect insulin secretion and disturb the whole symphony of hormonal balance in the human body.

5 Sugars, from glucose and sucrose to high-fructose corn syrup, are monumentally harmful. This is not only because the combination of fructose and glucose elevates insulin levels, but because it also overloads the liver.

6 Consuming excess calories does not cause us to grow fatter. Nor does expending more caloric energy than we consume lead to long-term weightloss. It only creates hunger.

7 Because of the effect that grains, cereals, starchy vegetables and sugars have on insulin, they are triggers in the development of diabetes and coronary heart disease. They are also major contributors to cancer, Alzheimer's disease and the other diseases of civilization, including premature ageing.

8 Gaining fat and being unable to get rid of it are the result of an imbalance, a disequilibrium in the hormonal regulation of fat tissue and fat metabolism. When hypothalamic regulation is not functioning correctly, the build-up of adipose tissue and the storing of fat exceeds the mobilization of fat from the body and we become obese. When hormonal regulation and hypothalamic balance are restored, this reverses the process and we can shed our inessential fat deposits.

9 Grains, cereals, sugars and starchy vegetables increase hunger and decrease the amount of energy expended through metabolism and physical activity.

10 Because carbohydrates have such a powerful effect in stimulating insulin secretion, they are the major cause of obesity. The fewer grain-based, cereal-based, sugar-based carbohydrates we consume, the leaner we will be for ever.

Safe or Not?

One question remains to be answered. Is a diet that is mostly or completely lacking in cereal-based, grain-based, sugar-based carbohydrates a healthy way of eating? For more than fifty years we have been told that it is not. Yet the most dramatic alteration in human diet in the past two million years has been the transition from a carbohydrate-poor to a carbohydrate-rich diet, which took place during the agricultural revolution as grains and starchy vegetables were added to the diet of our hunter-gatherer ancestors. Then why do most so-called experts in nutrition still insist that we should eat 120–130g of carbohydrates a day?

This figure was arrived at some time ago because this is the quantity of glucose that the central nervous system and brain will metabolize when someone is eating a diet rich in grain-based, cereal-based, sugar-based carbohydrates. The catch is this: what the nervous system and brain *use* and what they *need* are two different things. Without these carbohydrates in the diet, both the nervous system and the brain run perfectly well on *ketone bodies*, as did those of our Palaeolithic ancestors.

Brain foods

The body creates ketone bodies out of the fats we eat and from the fatty acids released from our adipose tissue. Our brain and nervous system also run on glucose, which our body has converted from the proteins that we eat, as well as on glycerol released from fat tissue in the form of triglycerides which are turned into free fatty acids. And, since a diet low in grain-based, sugar-based, cereal-based carbohydrates contains good quantities of fats and proteins and vegetable carbohydrates, there is never going to be a shortage of fuel for the nervous system or the brain. In fact, there is mounting evidence that these are likely to be the perfect fuels for our brain and our nervous system – the ones on which our bodies have evolved to run.

Nevertheless, the doctrine that 120–130g of carbohydrate per day is needed continues to reign supreme, sometimes with amusing effects. A report called *Dietary Reference Intakes*, issued by the Institute of Medicine (IOM) in the United States in 2002, acknowledges that the brain functions perfectly without carbohydrates because it runs superbly well on ketone bodies, glycerol and protein-derived glucose. It's absurd, then, that the report continues to insist that the 'recommended dietary allowance' of carbohydrate is 130g. How long such dogma will continue to govern people's beliefs about food is anybody's guess. As far back as 140 years ago the *Lancet* reported that 'the sugar and starchy elements of food' – that is, the cereal, grain and sugar carbohydrates – are what cause fattening and obesity. Meanwhile, the rest of the world goes on believing that gaining and losing weight depends on nothing more than willpower and that it's all a question of calories in, calories out.

End Obesity For Ever

In the so-called civilized world, human beings are fatter than ever. What's worse, we grow fatter still with each year that passes. Food manufacturers, government bodies and well-meaning doctors urge us to eat bread and cereals, rice and pasta. Meanwhile, extensive research into the effect of such fare on insulin resistance, obesity and the development of degenerative diseases shows quite clearly that these are precisely the foods that have made us fat in the first place. Apart from the fact that it can take a century for research to impact on health, much of the refusal to recognize what this kind of eating is doing to ruin our shape and our health comes not so much from 'ignorance is bliss' as 'ignorance is profitable'.

Food manufacturers long ago latched on to the notion that lots of carbs and low fat were supposed to be good for you. They were quick to translate fat-free, low-fat and reduced-fat dogma into huge profits. For twenty years the convenience-food market has been flooded with low-fat biscuits, muffins, cheeses, sweets and 'energy bars'. Virtually all of them are riddled with sugar – all superbly effective for anyone who wants to get fatter. The fat that food processors remove from these low-fat foods goes into making sweet treats and chocolate which are then sold to us on TV as goodies which we should eat if we really 'love ourselves'.

The humorist P. J. O'Rourke has pointed out that the world is now full of 'masses waddling into airports, business offices and churches dressed in drooping sweats or fuchsia warm-up suits or mainsail-size Bermuda shorts, each with a mobile phone in one ear and a Walkman in the other and sucking diet Pepsi through a straw.' All thanks to low-fat-high-carb dogma.

The bottom line is this: if you want to maintain the new, lean body that you've been given on Cura Romana, you will need to minimize grains and cereal-based carbohydrates and sugars. You may need to cut them out completely.

If, like me, you always have to get to the bottom of something and you want to understand more about how we get fat and how distorted the information we get through the media and so-called scientific studies is, you could not do better than to pick up a copy of *Good Calories, Bad Calories* by Gary Taubes, published by Alfred A. Knopf in 2007. Taubes is one of the finest researchers I have ever encountered when it comes to sorting truth from fiction in relation to diet, health, insulin resistance and obesity. He spent many years writing the book, which deals in great detail with many of the issues you find in this chapter. It is an excellent source of clear, unbiased information, complete with a bibliography so complete it may make your head spin. One word of warning however: although the book is not difficult to read, it is not for the faint-hearted since it deals in great depth and complexity with these issues.

People vary tremendously in how much of various grain-based, cereal-based carbohydrates they can handle. Some can cope with very little indeed and are better off leaving them out of their diet altogether. Others can eat small quantities of grains and cereals, as well as sugars. You need to find out from your own body – and there is no greater opportunity to do this than while you are in Consolidation. Once you do, you will have choices to make. On these choices will depend how much you value your leaner body and how much you want to continue to enhance your health for the rest of your life.

Forget Fat-free

For generations we have been told that fat is unhealthy. Don't you believe it. Many false beliefs surround fats. Your body's tissues, hormones and all its cells are dependent for their health on a good supply of essential fats. If you don't get enough of these (and almost nobody does on a low-fat regime), your overall health is compromised and you age more rapidly. But they need to be the right kind of fats.

Fat-free and low-fat diets cause your body to age prematurely. They create sub-clinical fatty-acid deficiencies. So do diets high in junk fats – margarines, ready-made salad dressings and sauces, convenience foods and the golden vegetable oils you see lined up on supermarket shelves, which many still claim are supposed to be good for us. On a typical Western diet, where 45 per cent of our calories come from fats, fatty-acid deficiencies are rampant. Why? Because your body cannot make use of the trans-fatty acids – or 'junk fats' – in the foods you are eating. Here are only a few of the conditions that result from a fatty-acid deficiency: premature ageing, heart disease, suppressed immunity, PMS, arthritis, dry skin, raised cholesterol levels and emotional and behavioural problems.

What is a fat?

Fat is a macro-nutrient which exerts little effect on your insulin levels, but which strongly decreases your appetite. Provided you are getting the right kind of fats in your diet, they can rejuvenate and balance your hormone levels and re-orientate how you look and feel, thanks to their effects on important regulatory chemicals called prostaglandins. Organic compounds scientifically known as triglycerides, all fats are composed of a glycerol molecule with fatty acids connected to it. Chemically, a fatty acid consists of a chain of carbon and hydrogen atoms to which one oxygen atom is attached. A molecule of fat differs from a molecule of carbohydrate (which is also made of carbon, hydrogen and oxygen) because the fat molecule contains a lot less oxygen. This is what makes fat highly concentrated and why there are 9 calories to each gram of fat you eat but only 4 calories to each gram of carbohydrate or protein. Incidentally, we tend to think that a 'calorie' is a bad thing. A calorie is just the measurement used to describe the energy-producing value of foods.

Scientists divide fats roughly into two groups – saturated and unsaturated. A saturated fat is a fatty acid with a molecule in which each carbon atom is connected to a hydrogen atom. This means there are no empty spaces to allow one or more of its carbons to reach out and join together with molecules of other substances. Because of this, saturated fats – found in meat, dairy products like cheese, ice cream, milk and tropical oils like palm kernel oil and coconut oil – are stable, relatively inactive and virtually inert in your body. There are exceptions to this, however, which we will look at in a minute. The *raison d'être* for most saturated fats is to provide energy that can be stored in your body's fat cells, especially in times of famine, to be used later.

The second group of fats, the unsaturates, are very different. They are mostly found in foods of vegetable origin like nuts and seeds, grains and avocados, although some of the most important omega-3 oils are also found in fish and game. Unlike saturated fats, such as butter, which are solid, unsaturated fats come in liquid form.

According to classical nutrition, only two unsaturated fatty acids are necessary for human health – linoleic and alpha-linolenic acids. Out of these two, your body is supposed to be able to make all the other fatty acids it needs. The trouble is that many people, having lived for years on commercial foods, lose their ability to make conversions. They need to get their fatty acids in a more direct way.

Essential fatty acids are vital because they are the fundamental nuts and bolts that your body uses to structure the brain, eyes, ears, reproductive organs and cell membranes that surround and protect every cell in your body. Without them you would not be able to move a muscle. You could not think, see or hear. Essential fatty acids are also needed for your body to make the hormone-like chemicals called prostaglandins. Critical to cellular functioning in the body, a good balance of prostaglandins helps your body resist illness – from arthritis and ulcers to migraines and cancer. It also supports the functions of your immune system, reproductive system, central nervous system and heart. Finally, prostaglandins regulate your brain chemicals – neuro-transmitters – themselves created out of essential fatty acids. When their balance is good you thrive and are protected from inflammatory conditions, including rheumatic problems as well as a trigger-happy immune system.

Get the essentials

The omega-3 group of fats and the omega-6 group make up the essential fatty-acid group of fats. Head of the omega-3 family is alpha-linolenic acid. Head of the omega-6 family is linoleic acid. Palaeopathologists have determined that our distant ancestors consumed these essential fats in a ratio of between 1:1 and 3:1 omega-6 to omega-3. In other words, these essential fats were eaten in relatively equal quantities compared to the balance we get now. This, scientists believe, is an ideal balance. In modern times, the balance between our omega-6s and omega-3s has become completely screwed up. We now consume a ratio of omega-6 to omega-3 about 22:1 – far too high for optimal health.

Essential fatty acids do some wonderful things for the body. They:

- ensure insulin sensitivity and good blood-glucose control
- the omega-3s create natural appetite control
- reduce excessive inflammation
- regulate cholesterol levels, triglyceride levels and blood pressure
- maintain cellular hydration
- build good semi-permeable cell walls for beautiful, well-hydrated skin and healthy arteries
- enhance good prostaglandin production
- protect the myelin sheaths around nerve cells in the brain

Natural appetite control

The omega-3 fats are particularly good satiety nutrients. These natural appetite suppressants work in an interesting way. They release a hormone called cholecystokinin (CCK) from the stomach when you eat them. This hormone signals to your brain, letting it know that you feel satisfied. When you reduce the level of fat in a meal, your brain does not receive the same message and – although you may be filled with food – you still want to eat more. This is a common experience for people who sit down to a meal and, no matter how much they eat, still crave food at the end of it. This can lead to eating disorders and a real mistrust of your body and yourself, where you feel you have to watch yourself carefully lest your eating get out of hand. Add enough good-quality essential fatty acids – especially the omega-3 fish oils – to your diet and you gradually begin to feel full and satisfied. You also learn that you can trust your body's messages. Rich in omega-9 fats, olive oil contains oleic acid, a monounsaturated oil that is more resistant to the denaturing effects of heat and light than polyunsaturated oils. While omega-9 fats are not essential to the body, olive oil has many health-enhancing properties. Use it often in your salads and for wok-frying foods.

YOUR BODY SPEAKS

HAVING COMPLETED hCG+Food Plan, I hope you are beginning to look upon your body as a best friend. If so, Consolidation is set to become a life-changing passage for you. Consolidation guides you, consciously and systematically, to establish new ways of eating that strengthen your body as well as your self-worth, so that the emotional and spiritual expansion which began during hCG+Food Plan can become a way of life. The sensitive instrument within you which will enable you to identify the foods your body loves and the foods it hates is often referred to as your *second brain*.

Leslie's Mistake

Let me tell you a little story about what happened to me so you will understand what I'm talking about. Not long ago I came across a beautiful piece of organic Camembert. I bought it, then ate it with glee. It was delicious. The next day I found myself plunged into a state of exhaustion and depression. Nothing seemed to work properly. I also discovered I had gained more than 2 pounds overnight. The physical and mental confusion went on for another 24 hours before it cleared.

The only good thing about this unpleasant drama was that it reminded me of something that I've known for ages but had totally forgotten.

Unknowingly, what I had done was eat a food which my body didn't want and therefore could not handle well. I had expected it to be good for me – after all, it was organic and yummy. But no. The message my body sent me was direct and simple: 'Don't eat this food again if you want to maintain your vitality, emotional balance, mental clarity and lean body.' Thanks to my body's response to the Camembert, I got the message loud and clear. The message came from my gut – the second brain, which is located in the gut.

The Camembert incident made me laugh, since I should have known better. After all, I had learned about food sensitivities way back in the mid-1970s at the age of twenty-five, when I was privileged to participate in research that my friend Dr Richard Mackarness was doing at Basingstoke District Hospital. A physician of great vision and author of many books, including *Not All in the Mind*, Mackarness fought for, and single-handedly achieved, the recognition of 'clinical ecology' as a medical discipline in Britain. He and his colleagues had established that food intolerance, food sensitivities and food allergies can cause a variety of illnesses. I suspect you can guess what is right up there at the top of the list: obesity.

Your Second Brain

Your digestive system is, in truth, a second brain. It boasts as many nerve endings as your brain itself. When we eat foods that antagonize these nerve endings, we experience all sorts of physical and emotional states that hold us back. In the late 1970s and 1980s a number of published reports showed how people with disturbances in their gut often exhibit extreme symptoms, from disorientation and blunted judgement to deep fatigue, depression, slurred speech, confusion and delirium. More recently, researchers in Norway, and Carl Reitjeld and Dr William Straw of Great Plains Laboratory in the United States, demonstrated that a similar relationship exists between autism and dietary peptides.

No matter how well we eat or how good the quality of the foods we choose, our bodies have certain foods that they love and foods that they hate. This does not mean that some sinister pathology is at work in our system. Nor that you should race off to your doctor for 'food allergy' testing. Food allergy testing is notoriously inaccurate, by the way. Your body's preferences are nothing more than expressions of your unique genetic, biochemical and physiological make-up.

What Works for You

As you are beginning Consolidation, this is the time to discover the foods that work for your body and those that don't. You achieve this by paying attention to what your body tells you and how it reacts to what you have eaten. To maintain good energy and your weightloss, and to continue to strengthen well-being, simply eliminate from your way of eating the foods that don't work. Later on – a few months down the road – you can, if you like, experiment to see if your body can handle some of these foods, provided you eat them only once in a while.

Loves and Hates

Here are a few questions you can ask when you suspect you have eaten a food that your body hates:

1 Has your weight increased suddenly?
2 Are you tired?
3 Have you been revisited by old food cravings?
4 Do you long for more of the food you ate?
5 Do you feel disorientated?
6 Are you depressed?

Food sensitivities and food intolerance were first identified back in the 1920s by the famous American allergist Dr Albert Rowe. Clinical ecologists insist that they are likely to be the most common cause of chronic fatigue, weight gain and depression. Rowe called the chronic fatigue which comes with eating the foods your body can't handle *allergic toxaemia*. Later, when he realized just how widespread negative food reactions were, he came to refer to the condition this caused as 'allergic tension-fatigue syndrome'.

Food sensitivities are different from food allergies, in which you are experiencing an immune reaction to some food with which you have come into contact. Yet they have a lot in common. Following in Rowe's footsteps, Theron Randolph, MD, another pioneer in the field of environmental medicine, charted a myriad emotional and physical symptoms which are either caused by or aggravated by eating foods with which the body can't cope. Randolph had worked with over 20,000 patients in a career that spanned sixty years. He published almost 400 scientific articles on his discoveries. He reported that people who react badly to a food develop maladaptive, physiological addictions to these foods. These include weight gain and depression. The negative way their body reacts to these foods turns into cravings and addictions.

Food sensitivities were once relatively uncommon. Now they have become so widespread that nutritionally trained doctors estimate that between 70 and 90 per cent of us in the Western world experience symptoms associated with food reactions, although few of us realize what is taking place. There are major reasons for this almost exponential rise in food reactions. First, our immune system is increasingly challenged by the presence of chemical and energetic pollution in the environment. Next, the massive consumption of convenience foods has rendered large segments of the population deficient in minerals and vitamins, which would otherwise have helped protect them from sensitivity reactions. Finally, the convenience foods on which most people live these days are chock-full of the foods highest on the reactive food list: milk products, wheat and other grains, junk fats and chemical additives. The body's enzymes, whose job it is to digest milk products and grains, and protect it from chemical pollution, therefore become gravely over-taxed.

Here lies the rub

People become addicted to a food to which their body reacts negatively without realizing that it is the very act of eating this food that has caused their addiction. Let me explain. When you are sensitive to a food or chemical, you react negatively to it on first contact. But if you eat or drink it again and again so that you are continually exposed to it, this negative reaction, together with the symptoms it produced, becomes 'masked'. It's like the alcoholic who feels OK so long as he has a drink in his hand. Then, when alcohol is withdrawn from him, he goes 'cold turkey' and feels terrible.

When you stop eating a food to which your body reacts negatively, WHAM – you get withdrawal symptoms. When you decide to go cold turkey – that is, to stop eating this food – you can experience uncomfortable withdrawal symptoms similar to those of the alcoholic deprived of his 'fix'. I have observed this phenomenon in some people right at the start of hCG+Food Plan – especially those who had been drinking a lot of coffee or diet sodas, or eating a lot of grain and sugar-based carbohydrates. Their symptoms often include no energy, a bad headache, depression and cravings. Happily, most of these cold-turkey reactions pass quickly and they emerge feeling surprisingly light and well. Many experts in clinical ecology insist that alcoholism and food reactions share a common cause, common triggers and a common biochemistry. Eliminate foods to which your own body is sensitive – those your body hates – and cravings and addictions disappear.

Common Addictive Foods

This allergy-cum-addiction is the hidden cause behind the 'eat one biscuit, eat the whole packet' syndrome.

1 Cereals and grains containing gluten: wheat, spelt, rye, oats, barley, Kamut, triticale and corn.

2 Milk products: low-fat and non-fat milk, cream, sour cream, yogurt, cheeses. (Butter works fine for most people and therefore doesn't require testing because it is a fat and not a protein). Most convenience foods contain hidden milk protein and casein – from bread and cereals to chips and protein bars. If your body does not handle milk well, be vigilant about any processed foods you choose to eat.

3 Eggs: a common food to which some people have a sensitivity.

4 Nuts and seeds: cashews, almonds, hazelnuts, Brazil nuts, peanuts.

5 Soy products, negative reactions to which are growing exponentially. More than 90 per cent of the soy now grown in the world has been genetically modified. Soy products less likely to cause negative food reactions are the fermented soy foods such as natto, miso or tempeh.

6 Other cereal and grain-based foods: corn, millet, quinoa, amaranth, teff, rice.

7 Beans and lentils: these foods contain carbohydrates called *glucosides* which are hard for humans to digest, but which the bacteria in the gut can digest with ease, causing gas and bloating. If you are vegetarian and feel you *must* eat these foods, take a digestive enzyme formula containing *glucoamylase* or *amyloglucosidase*, which helps to digest them.

How to Test for Reactions

During the first three weeks of Consolidation, the most important foods to find out about are eggs and the milk products, including yogurt and cheese, as well as soy products and the various nuts. Test each separately. You will not be testing the starchy vegetables, cereals, grains and sugars until the beginning of Week 4 of Consolidation. By then you will be an old hand at testing.

1 Allow your body to ease into Consolidation by eating only simple foods in the first week, such as those you had been eating on hCG+Food Plan, but with no restrictions on how much – good proteins, green vegetables, plus two or three pieces of fruit, for example. On Day 3 or 4 of the first week, if your body feels as though it's getting used to more food, you can start testing.

2 Decide what food you want to test first. Eggs might be a good place to start, or a milk product. Eat abundantly of this food at one meal. Then do not eat any more of it until 48 hours have passed. This will give you time to find out if it is a food that works for you or not.

3 Don't test another food until you have already found out whether the last food you have tested works for you or not. For instance, say you test eggs on a Thursday. You do not eat eggs on Friday. Nor do you test a new food until Saturday. By that time you will know about how your body gets on with eggs.

4 If it turns out that the first food you tested – eggs in this case – works fine for you, you can eat them as you like. You can then test a new food on Saturday – maybe Parmesan cheese – following the same testing procedures.

Food testing is not difficult once you get the hang of it. By the time the first couple of weeks of Consolidation are coming to an end, you will have a good idea about which foods work for you and which foods do not.

Not until Week 4 of Consolidation begins can you start testing the cereals, grains, starchy vegetables and sugars.

Identifying a bad reaction

As far as Cura Romana is concerned, here are the most common simple experiences to look for if you have eaten a food your body does not do well on:

1 Have your energy levels dropped for no apparent reason?

2 Has your weight gone up more than 2 pounds (900 grams) above the weight your body settled into on the first two or three days of Consolidation?

3 Are you craving certain foods or feeling ravenously hungry?

4 Are your bowels upset – constipation, gas or diarrhoea?

5 Do you feel emotionally unsettled for no apparent reason?

6 Have your spirits sunk for no apparent reason?

7 Do you have aches and pains in your body?

You are unlikely to experience all these things at once. You may only experience one or two. They will be your indicators.

How to handle a bad reaction

- Don't start thinking you have done something wrong. As Miles Davis said, 'Do not fear mistakes. There are none.'
- Give thanks to your body for telling you what doesn't work for you.
- Start drinking enough clean water or herbal tea to make you urinate frequently.
- If your reaction has been very strong, you might like to take a therapeutic dose of pure ascorbic acid – 2–4g every 3–4 hours until the reaction passes.
- Do a Steak Day (see page 225–6). Don't neglect this. It's important to correct the diencephalic reset. This will clear any weight gain that has taken place.
- When your reactions have dissipated and you start eating again, avoid the food or foods that have caused your body to react badly.
- Keep an ongoing record in your journal of all the foods your body loves and thrives on, which you can eat freely, as well as those foods it hates so you can avoid them in the future.

Reintroducing foods

This question usually comes up sooner or later: 'Will I *ever* be able to eat this or that food again?' After eliminating negative trigger foods from your diet for at least three months – six months is even better – you can try introducing first one and then another to see how your body handles them. If you eat them only now and then in small amounts, it may now be able to cope with them. However, if one or two of these foods represents a genuine 'food allergy' – coeliac disease, for instance – you will want to avoid them permanently.

A final note

Here are some suggestions to help you limit your reactive potentials long term.

- Choose what you eat from 'real' food rather than from packaged convenience foods. (And when I say 'real' food, I'm talking about food which nourishes us from seed to plate – which is grown or reared with a respect for human dignity and health, animal welfare, social justice and environmental sustainability.)
- Eliminate foods to which your body reacts negatively for between three and six months before trying them again.
- Read labels carefully to ensure that nothing you buy contains even minute quantities of the foods to which your body reacts negatively.
- Minimize your intake of grains and cereal products.
- Minimize your intake of dairy products (butter is OK) such as cheese, milk, yogurt, etc.
- Eat a large raw salad every day.
- Eat at least three portions of green vegetables each day.
- Eat two pieces of fruit each day.
- Eat ground flaxseeds and sprouted seeds.
- Eat baked or steamed oily fish two or three times a week – salmon, mackerel, halibut, sardines, herring.
- Drink 2 litres of liquids a day chosen from water, herbal teas and tea.
- Avoid coffee, fruit juices and any sweetened drinks.

Few people realize their full potential for radiant health, energy, clarity, emotional balance and creative power. To a far greater degree than most people realize, fatigue, brain fog, depression and weight gain result from their being unaware of the foods on which their body thrives and the foods with which it does not cope. Thanks to the health-enhancement, internal cleansing and renewed balance hCG+Food Plan brings, Consolidation is the perfect time for you to learn to make good choices. If you want to make your weightloss permanent, this simple food testing offers you the wherewithal to make it happen.

RULES OF THE GAME

Y OU HAVE PROBABLY been planning all the delicious things you are going to add to your diet now that Consolidation is beginning. That's great. But go easy during the first week. Stick to foods that are simply prepared. Don't mix too many things together, like grapes and cheese and nuts. Give yourself a chance to come to terms with the changes in your appetite which you will discover have taken place as the diencephalon rebalanced itself.

Remember too that you have been living on an oil-free diet for weeks now. So give your body a little time to adjust to the good-quality oils which you can begin to use from the very first day – olive oil, butter and coconut oil.

If you don't heed these warnings, you might end up creating biochemical and energetic chaos, the consequences of which can be bloating, diarrhoea, constipation, emotional upset, fatigue and, alas, rapid weight gain.

A Whole New World

At first Consolidation may seem a bit of a challenge. You've become accustomed to measuring your specific foods. Suddenly you have a wide variety of foods available and you have choices to make. From now on you will be learning how to play by your own body's rules. This is a time for learning what those 'rules' are and honouring them. There are two crucial weeks in Consolidation. Week 1, as your body is in transition from hCG+Food Plan, and Week 4, when you begin to introduce cereal-based and grain-based carbohydrates, starchy vegetables and sugars if you want to. Here is a brief outline of what Consolidation looks like:

1 Weigh yourself each morning And, if you travel, you must take your scales with you.

2 Eat simply in the first week Choose the same kind of foods you did on the Food Plan – simple proteins, vegetables and fruits. You may have as much or as little of them as feels right to you. Let your body dictate how much it wants day by day.

3 Weeks 1–3 Eat whatever foods you like in the quantities with which your body feels happy. However, you are not allowed to eat cereals, grains, flours, sugars, syrups, dried fruits, dates and raisins, or starchy vegetables like potatoes during the first three weeks. Save these until Week 4, when you can begin to test them.

4 Weeks 4–6 From Day 22 onwards you can gradually introduce grains, starchy vegetables and sugars, one by one. Testing is essential when it comes to introducing grain-based foods, flour and sugar-based foods and syrups.

Move gently into new ways

During the first week, go easy. Don't flood your system with too much food all at once. Increase the quantity and variety of foods step by step.

Simeons says: *Most patients are surprised how small their appetite has become and yet how much they can eat without gaining weight. They no longer suffer from an abnormal appetite and feel satisfied with much less food than before. In fact, they are usually disappointed that they cannot manage their first normal meal, which they have been planning for weeks.*

As soon as your body feels comfortable with the larger quantities of food, it's important to increase your protein intake. While on hCG+Food Plan you were living on minimal protein. This is the time to start rebuilding your protein stores. Now is also the time to return to taking a multivitamin or other supplements if you want to. What surprises many people who were big supplement-takers is that now they don't seem to want anywhere near as many nutritional supplements as they once did.

To Breakfast or Not to Breakfast?

Tune in and follow the messages of your unique body. For example, do you eat breakfast every morning or do you not? We have been taught that it's essential to eat breakfast. Breakfast should be the big meal of the day, should it not? Perhaps – but for you, this may not be true. I've been surprised to discover that more than half of people moving into Consolidation prefer not to eat breakfast every day. They tell me they feel great in the morning. They say that they love the sense of freedom and clarity they found during Cura Romana. They prefer not to put food into their bodies until lunchtime. So they choose to have breakfast or brunch only occasionally, often shared with good friends. There is no 'right' or 'wrong' to all this. So experiment and find out what works best for you.

Weigh Yourself Each Morning

During Consolidation, it is imperative that you continue to weigh yourself every morning as you have been doing. Minor variations in weight of between 1 and 2 pounds are normal at the start. Within the first few days after finishing the hCG, your weight is likely to settle at a pound or so above or below the final weight on your last day of the Food Plan. I call this your 'median weight'. If one day you wake up to find you have gained even a tiny bit more than 2 pounds – 900 grams – above this median weight, you can be sure that your body is giving you some important information: either something you have eaten, a mixture of foods you have taken together, or possibly eating more food at one time than your body wanted. This is the time to correct it by doing a Steak Day.

> **Simeons says:** *As long as their weight stays within two pounds of the weight reached on the day of the last injection, patients should take no notice of any increase; but the moment the scale goes beyond two pounds, even if this is only a few ounces, they must on that same day entirely skip breakfast and lunch but take plenty to drink. In the evening they must eat a huge steak with only an apple or a raw tomato. Of course this rule applies only to the morning weight. Ex-obese patients should never check their weight during the day, as there may be wide fluctuations and these are merely alarming and confusing.*

I have never been able to figure out why Simeons' Steak Days work so well – yet they do. Not only do they quickly bring your weight down to where it was, but, even more importantly, they protect the hypothalamus, pituitary and thalamus in the diencephalon from any tendency they may still have to return to the distorted functioning that was a major reason you were overweight before Cura Romana.

> **Simeons says:** *It is of utmost importance that the meal is skipped on the same day as the scale registers an increase of more than two pounds and that missing the meals is not postponed until the following day. If a meal is skipped on the day in which a gain is registered in the morning this*

brings about an immediate drop of often over a pound. But if the skipping of the meal – and skipping means literally skipping, not just having a light meal – is postponed the phenomenon does not occur and several days of strict dieting may be necessary to correct the situation.

The longer your body stays within a very small range of weight after hCG+Food Plan – from half a pound to a pound above or below your median weight – the quicker your body consolidates your new weight set point and the more healthily it continues to function. If you allow yourself to gain more than 2 pounds, or if you forget to weigh yourself each day and don't realize what you are doing, it will be much harder to restore balance and functioning. If you delay making the correction for more than 48 hours, a small fixed deposit of fat begins to re-establish itself. This in turn sends messages to the weight-control centre in your brain, encouraging it to return to the way it was functioning before beginning Cura Romana. You don't want to let this happen.

How to Do a Steak Day

Skip breakfast and lunch, but drink plenty of fluids – 2–3 litres. For the evening meal (you can have this meal in the afternoon if you prefer) eat a huge steak – the biggest that you can manage – with only a delicious, juicy apple or a raw tomato to accompany it. If you don't eat meat, I have found that a large piece of salmon or fresh tuna steak works just as well. For strict vegetarians, a large omelette made from 4–6 whole eggs is the obvious choice. A double quantity of micro-filtered whey protein is also an option here, but omelettes work better.

Simeons says: *Most patients hardly ever need to skip a meal. If they have eaten a heavy lunch they feel no desire to eat their dinner, and in this case no increase takes place. If they keep their weight at the point reached at the end of hCG+Food Plan, even a heavy dinner does not bring about an increase of two pounds on the next morning and does not therefore call for any special measures.*

Plenty of Fibre

If you happen to eat more than your body is asking for during the first week – the transition period between hCG+Food Plan and Consolidation – you may become constipated. Consider using one of the senna teas you have been using in the past few weeks – just temporarily, never long term – or some other helper just to clear the constipation. Meanwhile, the best fibre in the world for human beings is the kind found in fresh raw vegetables. Eat as great a variety of them as you can. Flaxseeds sprinkled into smoothies, on salads or fruit salads, or turned into delicious flaxseed crackers are a good fibre source for most people. You can easily make your own at home (see page 256). I add a tablespoon of organic psyllium husks to a smoothie once a day. It gives the smoothie a lovely consistency – a bit like a frothy milkshake. Find out what works best for you. Be sure to drink plenty of clean water, either on its own or in the form of herbal teas; 2 litres a day is good. Larger and taller people are likely to need more, as are athletes. Continuing to drink water in this way helps maintain your weight, your health and the health of your digestive system all through Consolidation and beyond.

Raw Food

I am a great believer in the benefits of raw food, so it will come as no surprise that I recommend you should aim to eat half your foods raw. Raw foods have rejuvenating and regenerative powers. This is why they are used throughout the world at the most famous natural clinics and spas for beauty, as well as for healing chronic and acute illness. They improve cellular functioning, enhance the energy and biochemistry of your body, and provide high levels of antioxidant and immune-enhancing plant factors. They also help maintain the balance and cleanliness that you experienced on hCG+Food Plan.

The Story of Wine

As soon as your body has settled into the first week of Consolidation – usually by Day 3 or 4 – you can enjoy a glass of wine with a meal once a day. As for high-carbohydrate foods, don't touch them until Week 4. Only then is your body stable enough to begin to test these foods.

Simeons says: *It takes about 3 weeks before the weight reached at the end of the treatment becomes stable. During this period patients must realize that the so-called carbohydrates, that is sugar, rice, bread, potatoes, pastries etc, are by far the most dangerous. If no carbohydrates whatsoever are eaten, fats can be indulged in somewhat more liberally and even small quantities of alcohol, such as a glass of wine with meals, does no harm; but as soon as fats and starch are combined things are very liable to get out of hand. This has to be observed very carefully during the first 3 weeks after the treatment is ended otherwise disappointments are almost sure to occur.*

The wine issue is a fascinating one. The worst worry for some people as they get ready to begin Cura Romana is: 'How am I going to live without my glass of wine at the end of the day?' To my amazement, many of those who most loved wine before they started the programme report afterwards: 'Strange, but I no longer seem to like wine very much.'

Suggested Foods from Week 1 Onwards

The lists of foods below gives you some suggestions of foods to eat on Consolidation.

GREAT CHOICE PROTEINS		
Meat and Poultry (lean, organic)	beef lamb pork veal	chicken lamb's liver turkey
Game Meats	venison rabbit other wild game	wild goat hare
Eggs (free-range)	whole eggs	egg whites
Fish and Seafood (sustainably sourced, preferably wild)	bass cod* crayfish halibut lobster mussels (green-lipped) prawns sardines* shrimps squid/calamari tuna steak* * rich in omega-3 essential fatty acids	clams crab haddock John Dory mackerel* oysters salmon* scallops snapper swordfish trout*

Protein-rich Dairy Foods (eat only occasionally)	Cheddar feta Parmesan	cottage cheese goat's cheese sheep's/ewe's milk cheese
Nuts (eat small quantities)	almonds hazelnuts walnuts	cashews macadamia

GREAT CHOICE CARBOHYDRATES

Raw Vegetables	alfalfa sprouts (and other sprouted seeds) bamboo shoots cabbage celery endive fennel lettuce onions radishes salsa spinach	broccoli cauliflower cucumber escarole lamb's lettuce mushrooms peppers, sweet (capsicum) rocket snow peas
Cooked Vegetables	artichoke aubergine (egg plant) bok choi Brussels sprouts cauliflower kale mushrooms onions spinach turnip	asparagus beans, green broccoli cabbage courgette leeks okra sauerkraut Swiss chard/silver beet
Fresh Fruit	apple avocados blueberries cantaloupe honeydew melon lemon	apricots blackberries boysenberries grapefruit kiwi fruit lime

	mandarin	nectarine
	orange	peach
	pear	plum
	raspberries	strawberries
	tangerine	

FATS

Good Choices	almond butter
	butter
	coconut oil
	flax oil (organic, cold-pressed)
	olive oil
	olive oil and vinegar dressing
	olives

Poor Choices	golden oils, such as:	
	canola	margarine
	peanut	safflower
	sunflower	

Suggested Foods from Week 4 Onwards

On Day 22 you will be entering the second critical week of Consolidation. This is the time when you will want to call on your practical food-testing skills to find out how well you deal with some of the high-glycemic carbo-hydrate foods – grains, cereals, starchy vegetables and sugars. A few people appear able to cope easily with some of these foods – perhaps 15 per cent do. Another 20–30 per cent of participants find that they can handle only a few of these foods and need to avoid the rest. The majority, however, report that they prefer to live without them altogether, except in small quantities and only occasionally. Your job is to find out which group you fit into. Most people get on well with both kasha (buckwheat) and wild rice – neither of which is a grain, but a seed.

STARCHY CARBOHYDRATES – TAKE CARE

Starchy Vegetables	acorn squash	baked beans
	beetroot	black beans
	broad beans (fava beans)	butternut pumpkin
	carrot	corn
	green beans	kidney beans
	lentils	lima beans
	parsnips	peas
	pinto beans	potato, baked
	potato, boiled	potato, chips or crisps
	potato, mashed	re-fried beans
	string beans	sweet potato
	white beans	
Grains, Cereals and Breads	bagel	biscuits
	breadcrumbs	bread, wholegrain
	bulgar wheat	cake
	cereal	chickpeas
	cornflour	couscous, dry
	crackers	croissant
	crouton	doughnut
	English muffin	granola
	lentils	millet
Condiments	barbecue sauce	cocktail sauce
	honey	ice cream
	jam or jelly	molasses
	plum sauce	relish, pickle
	sugar	sugar, icing
	sweets	syrup, golden

The 12-point Plan for a Leaner Body

These eating guidelines work for the vast majority of people I have worked with on Cura Romana, both for Consolidation and for after. Each of us is utterly unique so, while the general principles are sound, it is up to you to discover what your own relationship to a specific food is.

1 Choose the foods you eat for two reasons: because they are irresistibly delicious and because, when you have eaten them, your body feels good afterwards. Be sure to keep careful day-by-day records of your meals and how you react to different foods.

2 Even during Week 4 (from Day 22 onwards), when you are allowed to begin introducing starches and sugars, try eating very few grain-based or plant-based carbohydrate foods, including cereals, flours and gravies made from them.

3 Eat as much as your body tells you to of natural, fresh, organic, non-starchy vegetables and low-sugar fruits (see chart, page 230). Non-starchy vegetables high in phytonutrients and antioxidants should be your primary source of carbohydrates.

4 Eat at least one gorgeous salad a day. Not the usual thing made from lettuce and tomatoes plus the odd cucumber, but a Cura Romana medley complete with a great variety of fresh herbs, crunchy sweet peppers and anything else fresh and beautiful that you can lay your hands on or grow on your kitchen windowsill.

5 Steer clear of soft drinks, packaged fruit juices, alcohol (except for a glass of good-quality wine a day, if you like).

6 Use cold-pressed, extra-virgin olive oil, walnut oil or flaxseed oil on salads, and coconut oil or olive oil for cooking. (Never heat flaxseed oil.) Butter is fine.

7 Enrich your diet with omega-3 fatty acids by eating fatty fish at least three times a week.

8 Stay away from margarine and other processed oils, such as peanut, sunflower and the other 'golden oils', and from any sauces or salad dressings that contain them.

9 Eat plenty of good-quality protein, like fresh fish, free-range chicken, eggs, game, organic meat, good micro-filtered whey and fermented soy foods if you are a vegetarian. Let your innate appetite be your guide.

10 Eliminate coffee, or at least drink only one cup a day.

11 Avoid packaged commercial foods as much as possible.

12 Right from the first week of Consolidation, eat half your foods raw, as raw foods have rejuvenating and regenerative powers. (See page 228 for more information on the benefits of eating raw foods.)

EAT FOR YOUR LIFE

PUT YOUR KITCHEN SCALES away and forget the complex routine for preparing a béchamel sauce. Now is the time to leave behind all the rules you may have learned before about what you should and shouldn't eat. From now on let your finely tuned body decide. It is not conventional directions that matter when preparing foods. It is a passion for the foods themselves – a feeling reflected in our passion for the earth and for life itself. You see it in a small child as he enthusiastically devours a bowl of fresh strawberries drizzled with honey. It's good because it tastes good. Such passion, which is visual, visceral and luscious, becomes the inspiration that, in food preparation, leads you automatically to make certain choices. If two things look good together they taste good together. You wouldn't put octopus and chicken in the same dish.

Open wide your kitchen window. Welcome the breezes of experiment, wit and spontaneity. Inside, you find the traditional meal of roast meat and boiled Brussels sprouts topped off with a piece of sticky toffee pudding replaced by something far more hedonistic: slivers of raw Pacific salmon, luscious garden-fresh salad, followed by a winter sorbet of cranberry and mint. Consolidation foods are lighter, richer in protein and full of texture, flavour and surprises. The real joy in eating fresh, light, protein-rich foods lies in their taste, their texture and the remarkable ability they have to bring excitement to a palate jaded by too many highly processed, unimaginatively seasoned or over-cooked dishes.

Sheer Energy

I love these recipes, first because they taste delicious, and second because together they make up a way of eating and living that supports the body with the highest levels of energy and well-being, not only while you are in Consolidation but ever after. I look on food as a source of both delight and life-energy which is passed on to us from the earth. I believe this energy needs to be preserved by not cooking food too much, by eating it fresh and by respecting its essential nature. Food eaten this way becomes a medium through which we build our own vitality – energy to protect the body from premature ageing and illness, to enhance good looks and to keep the mind clear. It is the life-energy present in abundance in fresh foods and the clean, simple protein from fish, game, organic meat and poultry that makes these foods irresistible and helps us look and feel great.

The most important foods for Consolidation and for the rest of your life are fresh non-starchy vegetables, fresh fruits, and proteins like meat, seafood, eggs and game. A little unprocessed cheese is fine too and a few nuts and seeds – provided, of course, you have checked these foods individually to make sure they work for your body. Go for nothing but the best. Here are some guidelines:

- Choose natural whole foods – organically grown/raised if possible.

- Your foods need to be as fresh as possible and eaten as close to a living state as you can. This allows little time for the deterioration that occurs as a result of oxidation.

- All the foods you eat should be non-toxic and non-polluting to your body. They should contain no synthetic flavours, colours, preservatives or other additives used to 'enhance' them cosmetically. Stay away from convenience foods.

- Try to vary the foods you choose from day to day and week to week. All through our evolution, the human body has adapted to a wide range of foods offering a broad spectrum of nutrients.

- Use fresh garlic and herbs often. They bring high-level support for cellular regeneration and immune support.

- Eat what you enjoy and enjoy what you eat. Eating is one of life's great pleasures – make it one of yours.

- When you discover what your body loves and what it doesn't handle, banish the latter from your life. As you do, the cravings you once struggled with will vanish and never return.

Full of life, phytonutrient power and just plain delicious, these fresh, living foods are the key to your thriving and remaining lean. Eat them often from now on.

Drinks

Continue to drink plenty of pure water. Buy it plain, sparkling or even naturally flavoured, so long as there are no artificial sweeteners added. Enjoy a wide selection of good herbal teas, green teas and white tea. Rich in antioxidants, white tea is the best drink around for health and weight maintenance.

Coffee, on the other hand, is a major contributor to tissue inflammation and blood-sugar disorders. Drunk in large amounts (more than one cup a day) it may disturb the new way the diencephalon area of your brain has been retrained on the programme. Coffee also dries out skin – even oily skin – making it prone to wrinkles. Avoid it altogether if you can. If not, limit yourself to one cup of organic coffee a day. You don't want coffee to undo all the good that Cura Romana has done for you.

- Use filtered or spring water. Do as Frenchwomen have done for decades – keep a large bottle or two of pure, fresh, mineral water within easy reach, and make sure you consume 8–10 big glasses daily.

- Drink white tea – either hot or cold.

- Enjoy herbal teas, flavoured mineral water (only those with no artificial sweeteners or calories) or sparkling mineral water.

- Try organic vegetable bouillon or broth. You can make your own broth with broccoli, cabbage, cauliflower, bean sprouts, asparagus, mustard greens, spinach, watercress, ginger, garlic or any such combination. Bring to the boil and simmer for 15 minutes. Season with herbs and sea salt and store in the fridge, reheating as needed.

Oils and Fats

Extra-virgin olive oil, cold-pressed flaxseed oil and walnut oil are best for salads. You can also use olive oil for wok-frying. Coconut fat is even better for this, and better than olive oil for searing meat or fish, since – being a saturated fat – it is highly stable. Coconut oil has some other important attributes too. It supports the thyroid, activates metabolism and is a fine source of just plain energy when you need it. It is also rich in medium chain triglycerides (MCT), which have been shown to reduce body fat, reverse arteriosclerosis, improve glucose metabolism and even lower serum and liver cholesterol.

The fats you want to eat on Consolidation are the healthiest available. Most can be used in salad dressings or for cooking proteins. Eat about a tablespoon or so per meal from the list below.

- avocados
- coconut oil
- extra-virgin olive oil
- macadamia nuts and macadamia butter
- olives
- tahini
- butter

About Snacks

Eat snacks only if you really feel the need. Most people find they feel better simply eating a couple of well-made meals a day. Here are some snack suggestions.

- a slice or two of chicken breast
- an apple, an orange, a pear or a few strawberries
- a small handful of unsalted walnuts, cashews, almonds or brazils
- a few crudités dipped in salsa
- a small amount of sunflower seeds
- a hard-boiled egg

Shopping

Sensuous, delicious meals begin at the shopping stage. Buy what's most beautiful. Forget the rest. It's time to leave packaged convenience foods behind to become part of your past, not of your future. Bring home meat and fish, eggs and salad vegetables. Wash your salad ingredients thoroughly and dry them, then place them ready to use in the vegetable compartment of your fridge. If you shop for fresh vegetables once or twice a week, do this as soon as you get home, then you are all set – not only for instant salads, but for instant whole meals.

Eat For Your Life Kitchen

The recipes which you find here are my own – developed and refined over many years. I have chosen my favourites to share with you. Some have appeared here and there in my previous books, such as *The Powerhouse Diet*. But all these recipes have continued to evolve into new incarnations. They are not only for use in part one and part two of Consolidation; I hope you will use your own variations on those you like long into the future. Some are suitable for the first three weeks of Consolidation, during which you are steering clear of starches and sugars; for others you must wait until Weeks 4, 5 and 6 before you try them out. Each recipe is carefully marked so you can tell which is appropriate to when.

Important note Do not assume that every recipe will be all right for you just because you find it here. For instance, if a recipe calls for eggs, or Parmesan cheese, you need to make sure the ingredients it contains belong to the list of foods your body loves and handles well, not to those it hates. Check the list of your body's loves and hates before using any of them. And don't hesitate to replace the Parmesan with fried tofu or grated hard-boiled egg when you come across an ingredient that your body does not handle.

All the Consolidation recipes that you find here have been tried and tested by Cura Romana participants who have given us feedback about what works best. They are not meant to be followed slavishly – they are here for inspiration. Use your creativity and experiment with them to develop even better ones. Food preparation is an art – not a science. Since high-raw is such a wonderful path to radiance and lasting leanness, let's look at salads first.

Salad secrets

The quickest and easiest way to stay lean and go on feeling as fabulous as you did on hCG+Food Plan is to make one meal a day a huge crunchy salad supported by good-quality protein – be it fish, chicken, eggs, tofu, seeds or nuts. We're talking rich green mesclun and brilliant flowers, wild herbs, fennel and orange with mangetout tendrils, bright sweet peppers, brilliant Swiss chard/silver beet and almonds – crisp, delicious and easy to make. Eat salads brimming with life-force and phytonutrients. This keeps your system clear, protects you from premature ageing and energizes your life. Salad-making is far more an art than a science. I am always amused by people who say they love salads but just don't have time to make them. I can create a salad as a whole meal for four people and have it on the table in under 10 minutes.

Wash and Bin

The key to keeping your vegetables fresh for a whole week once they've been washed is always to store them in plastic trays in the fridge and cover them with big plastic bags. When it comes to bunches of fresh herbs such as basil, coriander and parsley, I place them in a jug of cold water in the fridge. This way they too will last a week.

You can make a fabulous salad from a bunch of rocket and some gorgeous black olives, with fresh slivers of Parmesan cheese. You can make an entirely different salad from a beetroot and a couple of apples, grated using a mandolin, then dressed with fresh orange juice, a handful of chopped herbs and some curry powder. Delicious, nutrient-rich salads are simple to make. Use shredded raw broccoli and cauliflower, red and yellow sweet peppers, chopped red onion and slivers of Chinese leaves, smothered in a creamy home-made mayonnaise made with extra-virgin olive oil, or an irresistible curried avocado dressing.

Instrument of torture

The one piece of kitchen equipment I never want to be without is a mandolin. These remarkable vegetable-shredders are so different from the usual graters you find in most stores. Their tiny knives make perfect slices of whatever vegetable you like. You can julienne, make chip-size chunks, slice thin or thick. Unlike a conventional grater, which tends to mash vegetables and fruits, a mandolin slices clean and sharp.

Make it easy

Lazy about salad dressings, I usually make my salad in a large flat bowl. Then, instead of mixing the dressing separately, I dress the salad right there and then with a few tablespoons of extra-virgin olive oil, some chopped fresh herbs, crushed raw garlic, a dash of Worcestershire sauce, some Himalayan or Maldon sea salt, the juice of a lemon and a couple of tablespoons of apple cider or balsamic vinegar and some home-made cajun seasoning (see page 163). To top it off I use freshly ground black pepper. I like to grind peppercorns with a mortar and pestle because it tastes so much better that way. I sprinkle this all on top and toss. Ready in an instant. Sometimes I sprinkle salads with seeds like pumpkin, sesame or sunflower. At other times, I scatter with chopped fresh herbs or even fresh edible flowers like marigold petals, nasturtiums or heartsease.

Unleash Your Creativity

What you need to turn a simple salad into a masterpiece is a child's sense of experimentation, plus plenty of love. This is the secret ingredient that can make every meal you prepare a real joy. Putting together beautiful, brightly coloured gifts from nature becomes a kind of blissful meditation. What matters is not just what you make, or the ingredients you use, but your love of doing it, knowing that you are both honouring yourself and nurturing your own body as well as those of the people you are cooking for.

I often mix from two to five vegetables together to make a salad. Not only do I combine varieties of vegetables, I also mix textures, using fine julienned celeriac with a coarsely grated red cabbage, plus slivered spring onions. It's the mixture of colours and textures that makes it all work. Let imagination take over. Feel and taste the ingredients you are using. Treat the whole process of salad-making as you would that of painting a picture or making a sculpture. Have fun. Make it a delightful experience and you can't go wrong.

One bowl says it all

I love one-bowl eating. Maybe it is an atavistic regression to the ways of my peasant ancestors, but I love the idea of sitting down to a big salad, complete with top-quality protein – prawns or chicken, even tofu occasionally – all in one big bowl. One-bowls in any form consist of colourful, simple, tasty foods which are as good for you as they are delicious. They make a meal that is a pleasure to eat alone or to share with others. Once you get into creating one-bowl meals, you may wonder why you ever did anything else.

SNACKS, BREAKFASTS AND BRUNCHES

Live Muesli

serves 1

vegetarian

Good for all six weeks of Consolidation, but be sure to test for sensitivity to yogurt and nuts if you use them.

This is my own invention and my favourite muesli. It takes advantage of the health-enhancing properties of coconut oil. Everybody loves live buckwheat muesli – even children raised on sugar-crunch convenience foods. Not only are live mueslis higher in essential nutrients than their grain-based counterparts, but the quality of the phytochemicals they contain is the best in the world. This recipe calls for an apple, but you can use almost any fruit – strawberries, peaches, apricots, cherries, pears – whatever is inexpensive and in season. This version is dairy-free. If you prefer to use dairy products, you can use plain yogurt in place of the almond/rice milk. The raw buckwheat has been soaked overnight so that enzymes break down the hard-to-digest starches, making it taste sweeter while being much easier to absorb. It is even better if you let the buckwheat sprout for two or three days before you use it.

WHAT YOU NEED

2 tablespoons raw buckwheat, soaked overnight in water or sprouted for a day or two

2 teaspoons coconut oil – it is usually hard at room temperature (optional)

1 apple or any other fruit, chopped or grated

juice of 1 orange or tangerine

stevia, to taste

120ml almond milk, rice milk or yogurt (ensure there is no sugar or malt added to any of these)

1/2 teaspoon ground cinnamon or nutmeg, or some freshly grated ginger

HERE'S HOW

Mix together the soaked buckwheat with the coconut oil, using a fork to cream it all together. Combine with the fruit and juice, stevia, almond/rice milk or yogurt. Sprinkle with cinnamon or ginger and serve immediately.

Fruitier Muesli

Substitute some fresh fruit juice, such as apple, orange or grape, for the almond/rice milk or yogurt. To thicken the juice, blend with a little fresh fruit in season such as pear or apple.

Summer Muesli

Add a handful of fresh or frozen strawberries, blackberries, boysenberries, raspberries or stoned cherries to the basic muesli.

Vanilla Nutmeg Smoothie
serves 1

Good for all six weeks of Consolidation, but test for sensitivity to eggs first.

This breakfast-in-an instant is based on the traditional eggnog that people drink at Christmas. In fact, the egg is optional – you can make the smoothie with or without. If you decide to put the egg in – I like to do this because it gives more flavour – make sure it is free-range or organic. You don't want to mess around with raw battery-laid eggs because of salmonella.

WHAT YOU NEED

200ml cold filtered or spring water

6 ice cubes

1–2 scoops natural or vanilla-flavoured micro-filtered whey protein

1 organic or free-range egg (optional)

1 teaspoon vanilla essence (the *real* thing – no sugar, preferably organic)

pinch of freshly grated nutmeg, to taste

stevia, to taste

1 heaped teaspoon organic psyllium husks (optional)

1 tablespoon flaxseeds (optional)

HERE'S HOW

Place all the ingredients in a blender and blend vigorously until combined. Be careful not to blend more than 20 seconds, however, as this can change the nature of the micro-filtered whey protein. Sprinkle a little extra grated nutmeg on top and serve immediately.

Scrambled Tofu

serves 1

vegetarian

Good for all six weeks of Consolidation, but test for sensitivity to cheese first.

Lighter and more delicate in texture than scrambled eggs, tofu works well for breakfast provided you season it richly – it has almost no flavour of its own. If you add a pinch of turmeric, you will create a 'vegan scrambled egg' in a rich yellow, just like the real thing.

WHAT YOU NEED

1 teaspoon extra-virgin olive oil

2 green onions, finely chopped

2 cloves garlic, crushed or chopped

200g tofu

pinch of turmeric (optional)

Mexican chilli powder, to taste

1/2 teaspoon curry powder

1/2 teaspoon cumin powder

60g grated Parmesan (optional for vegetarians)

Himalayan or Malvern salt, to taste

freshly ground black pepper, to taste

HERE'S HOW

Heat the oil in a heavy frying pan and sauté the onions and garlic until they are soft (2–3 minutes). Mash the tofu, then stir it into the pan with the turmeric. Add the other spices and any other herbs you want. Cook over high heat, turning frequently, until the tofu is firm – about 2–3 minutes. Sprinkle on the cheese if you are using it. Season with salt and pepper and serve immediately.

Light-as-Air Pancakes

serves 2

vegetarian

Good for all six weeks of Consolidation, but test for sensitivity to cottage cheese and eggs first.

This is a recipe I developed for my family long before I was aware of low-grain eating. I used to make masses of it on Sunday mornings and my kids loved them. It makes very light and fluffy pancakes, rather like pancake soufflés. They need to be eaten immediately. The egg white that gives them their fluff gets lost quickly once they have been cooked. They can be served with a beautiful raspberry syrup recipe which can also be made with strawberries or blueberries (see page 248), some butter or some sugar-free jam.

WHAT YOU NEED

4 eggs

100g creamed cottage cheese

2 tablespoons soda water

Himalayan or Malvern salt, to taste

30g gram flour (besan/chickpea flour)

1/2 teaspoon baking powder

pinch of stevia, to taste

1–2 tablespoons coconut oil

HERE'S HOW

Separate the eggs and beat the whites until almost stiff. In another bowl, combine the egg yolks with the cottage cheese, soda water, salt, flour, baking powder and stevia. Blend thoroughly. Gently fold in the egg whites. Heat the coconut oil in a skillet or crêpe pan and spoon in individual dollops of the mixture, tilting the pan so that the mixture covers the bottom. Cook until the underside turns a light golden brown. Flip each pancake only once, cooking the second side until it is lightly browned. Remove from the heat. Serve immediately topped with butter and berry syrup or sugar-free jam.

Raspberry Syrup

serves 4

Good for all six weeks of Consolidation.

This you can also make with blueberries, strawberries, loganberries or blackberries – whatever happens to be in season. It's great on pancakes or cottage cheese for breakfast, or over Mascarpone as a dessert or snack.

WHAT YOU NEED

240g raspberries or other berries
120ml filtered or spring water
1 teaspoon grated orange or lime zest
stevia, to taste
pinch of ground nutmeg

HERE'S HOW

Put the berries in the water, bring to the boil and simmer gently over low heat. Add the other ingredients and cook very gently until the syrup thickens slightly, then remove from the heat. Either you can purée this syrup in a blender or you can leave it chunky and serve it as it is. It will keep well in the fridge for a week.

SALADS

Spinach, Egg and Mushroom Salad

serves 4
vegetarian

Good for all six weeks of Consolidation, but test for sensitivity to eggs first.

If you need to pack a lunch, this salad travels well provided you carry the dressing and the grated hard-boiled eggs in separate containers and add them just before serving.

The combination of spinach with grated hard-boiled eggs and mushrooms is a surprising one. The crunchiness of the spinach is offset by the rich, creamy protein properties of the eggs.

several large handfuls of baby spinach or very fresh full-grown
   spinach

1 cup raw white button mushrooms, washed and sliced

2 cloves garlic, finely chopped (optional)

120ml vinaigrette dressing

6 hard-boiled eggs, grated with a coarse grater

1/2 teaspoon red peppercorns (you can use black peppercorns if you
   don't have red ones)

HERE'S HOW

Clear out any wilted bits or nasty stalks from the spinach and give it a
really good wash, making sure to remove any soil. Spin it dry or dry it
in a tea towel, then pop it in the fridge for 15–20 minutes to crisp up.
When you're ready to serve, place the spinach leaves in a bowl, add the
mushrooms and sprinkle garlic over the top if using. Pour the
vinaigrette dressing over, top with grated hard-boiled eggs and
sprinkle with coarsely ground pepper. Serve immediately.

Chef's Salad

serves 2

Good for all six weeks of Consolidation, but test for sensitivity to eggs
and Parmesan first.

*A chef's salad is one of those perfect meals you can not only order in a
restaurant but also make yourself – provided you have plenty of left-
overs.*

WHAT YOU NEED

1 head of the most beautiful lettuce you can find (any kind), torn
   into bite-sized pieces

1/2 cucumber, cubed

1 tomato, cubed

3 tablespoons fresh parsley, basil or coriander, chopped

2 tablespoons lemon juice

2 tablespoons extra-virgin olive oil, or half olive oil and half flaxseed oil

1 teaspoon balsamic or apple cider vinegar

dash of Worcestershire sauce

2 cloves garlic, crushed or finely chopped

4 hard-boiled eggs, halved

100g cooked chicken, sliced in strips

100g ham, sliced in strips

50g Parmesan (or more, if you like it as much as I do), shaved

HERE'S HOW

Arrange lettuce, cucumber and tomato in a big flat salad bowl and sprinkle with the fresh herbs. Combine the lemon juice, olive oil, vinegar, Worcester sauce and garlic to make a dressing. Pour this over the salad and toss. Arrange the eggs, chicken, ham and cheese on top and serve immediately.

Grilled Prawns and Rocket Salad
serves 4 generously
meat-free

Good for all six weeks of Consolidation.

There is some magic about grilled prawns and rocket mixed together. The richness of the prawns and the crunchiness of the rocket – especially if you can get wild rocket – is worth any amount of effort to put together. The lovely thing about this salad is that it's no effort to make. You can grill the prawns ahead of time, then simply take them out of the refrigerator and add to the rocket, or you can grill them, as I tend to do, on a griddle or grill and serve them immediately on top of the rocket.

WHAT YOU NEED

400g tiger prawns

2 tablespoons extra-virgin olive oil

2 garlic cloves, chopped

zest and juice of 1/2 lemon

chilli flakes, to taste (optional)

Himalayan or Malvern salt, to taste

freshly ground red or black peppercorns

100 g rocket, washed and any heavy stems removed

vinaigrette dressing

HERE'S HOW

Peel the prawns and run a knife down their backs to pull away any small black threads. Rinse and pat dry. Heat the pan or grill, coating with a little olive oil. Cook the prawns quickly over high heat for about 3 minutes until they start to turn golden. While they're cooking, sprinkle them with garlic, lemon zest, chilli flakes, if using, salt and pepper.

Line a flat salad bowl with the rocket. The moment the prawns are done, remove them from the heat. Add a garlicky vinaigrette dressing, place the prawns on top and serve immediately.

Caesar Salad with Egg and/or Bacon Croutons
serves 4
meat-free, or not, as you like

Good for all six weeks of Consolidation, but check for sensitivity to eggs, bacon and cheese first.

Add something surprising to a salad – like egg and bacon 'croutons' – and do it your own way. Toss in slices of leftover chicken, fish or turkey to create a delicious whole meal in a bowl.

WHAT YOU NEED
2 heads romaine lettuce
12 anchovy fillets, drained and cut into thirds
50g Parmesan, shaved (not grated)

FOR THE CROUTONS
2 rashers lean bacon, diced, fried and drained (optional)
2 hard-boiled eggs, quartered

FOR THE DRESSING
juice of 3 medium-sized lemons
2 garlic cloves, finely chopped or crushed
4 tablespoons extra-virgin olive oil
several dashes of Worcestershire sauce
Himalayan or Malvern salt, to taste
freshly ground black pepper, to taste
1 free-range organic egg

HERE'S HOW
To prepare the dressing In a small bowl, mix together the lemon juice, garlic, olive oil, Worcester sauce, salt and pepper. Break the whole egg into the bowl and whisk with a fork to blend well.

To prepare the salad Wash and dry the lettuce leaves, then tear them into chunky morsels. Wrap them in a clean tea towel and chill in the fridge until you need them. Place the lettuce leaves in a large flat salad bowl, add the cooled 'croutons' and pour the freshly made salad dressing all over. Add the anchovies and season. Toss, then serve with shaved Parmesan.

California Sprouted Salad

serves 2

vegan

Good for all six weeks of Consolidation.

This salad relies heavily on sprouted seeds and grains. Sprouts are vegetables which grow in any climate, mature in 3–5 days, can be 'planted' any day of the year, need neither soil nor sunshine, and are some of the richest sources of antioxidant vitamins, minerals and phytonutrients in the world. Grow them in jars in your kitchen or in the airing cupboard. Buy them in the supermarket. They are the perfect compromise between the agriculture of years gone by and the 'just add water' mentality of the twenty-first century. Sprouts are also rich in chlorophyll, known to have anti-ageing properties.

WHAT YOU NEED
1 cup crunchy lettuce, mesclun, endive or spinach
1 tomato, sliced
1 tablespoon green onions, finely chopped
1 avocado, sliced
2 cloves garlic, crushed or chopped
1/2 bulb fennel, sliced
1/2 cup alfalfa sprouts
1/2 cup sunflower sprouts
Himalayan or Malvern salt, to taste
freshly ground pepper, to taste

HERE'S HOW
Wash and shred the greens and place in a serving bowl. Lay the tomato, onion and avocado over the lettuce, then add the garlic and fennel. Top the salad off with alfalfa and sunflower seeds, season and pour your favourite dressing over.

FLAX MAGIC

Few of us in the Western world ever seem to get enough quality fibre. The best in the world comes from fresh vegetables and sprouted seeds, but a good alternative is flax. You would be hard pressed to find any food that's higher in fibre – both soluble and insoluble. Flaxseeds – also known as linseeds – are high in most of the B vitamins, in magnesium and manganese. They are also very rich in omega-3 fatty acids.

When you enter Consolidation you are no longer bound by not being able to eat things that have oils in them. Omega-3 fatty acids are a key force against inflammation in the body. There is a lot of evidence to show that inflammation plays a very important part in many chronic diseases, including skin ageing itself, heart disease, arthritis, diabetes, asthma, etc. Flaxseeds are also a great source of phytochemicals, which help balance female hormones.

The fibre in flaxseed is primarily responsible for its cholesterol-lowering effect. Fibre helps stabilize blood sugar and, most important, it promotes the proper functioning of the bowels. This matters all the way through our lives. Unless our bodies get enough fibre, we do not eliminate wastes properly from our system and then we become much more susceptible to illness.

You can use flaxseeds in many different ways. You can mix them into smoothies, salads, yogurt or, if you are eating it, porridge. A wonderful way of being able to eat fun crunchy foods that are also good for you and get plenty of fibre at the same time is to make flaxseed crackers. They are delicious.

Flaxseed Crackers

vegan

Good for Weeks 2–6 of Consolidation.

You can make these in one or two ways. Either cook them in the oven or – if you happen to have a dehydrator or live in a country with masses of sunshine – you can make them raw, in effect, and dehydrate them. It's a good idea to grind up most of the flaxseeds (in a coffee grinder or food processor), because this releases more of the nutritious vitamins, minerals and phytochemicals that they contain. For a crunchier texture, leave a portion of the flaxseeds whole.

WHAT YOU NEED

240g flaxseed meal
240ml water
30ml tamari or Bragg's Liquid Aminos or soy sauce
Himalayan or Malvern salt, to taste
fresh minced herbs
a little garlic, chopped
ginger, chilli powder or cayenne pepper (optional)

HERE'S HOW

Combine the flaxseed meal with the water and let it soak for 1 1/2 hours. The water will change to a sort of gelatinous state. Check the mixture and add a little more water if necessary – you want it to be gooey but not runny and not too thick. Next add the tamari (or Bragg's or soy sauce), salt, some fresh minced herbs and a little garlic. You can also add a little ginger, chilli powder or cayenne pepper if you like. Blend together. Spread this mixture out, about 1/8 inch thick, on your dehydrator's Paraflex or Teflex sheets and set the dehydrator to about 110°F. Dehydrate for 4–6 hours, then turn the mixture over and dehydrate again for 3–4 hours. If you like crunchy crackers, dehydrate a bit longer. If you like them chewier, dehydrate them a bit less. Then break or slice them into pieces. These can also be baked in a slow oven – remove the crackers when they look done.

SEXY SAUCES

Winning Pesto
makes about 480ml
vegetarian

Good for all six weeks of Consolidation, but test for sensitivity to nuts and cheese first.

Probably my favourite sauce of all time is Italian pesto. I grew up eating it over pasta and for a time missed it terribly when I wasn't eating pasta. Then I realized that the same sauce, which is low-carb, goes brilliantly on fish, green beans, spaghetti squash – even a salad of buffalo Mozzarella and thinly sliced tomatoes. I make this sauce in a blender, store it in the fridge and use it within two days. I am notorious for buying huge bunches of fresh basil and making masses of pesto. When I want to freeze it, I make it without the cheese, then add the cheese when I defrost it. Pesto keeps very well this way.

WHAT YOU NEED
240ml extra-virgin olive oil
4–6 cloves garlic, crushed or chopped
a huge bunch of fresh basil leaves, about as much as you can gently
    pack into 3 big cups
70g pine nuts, macadamias or even almonds
70g freshly grated Parmesan

HERE'S HOW
Put the olive oil into a blender and add everything except the cheese. Blend until smooth. Pour into a bowl and stir in the cheese.

Hollandaise Sauce
serves 4
vegetarian

Good for Weeks 2–6 of Consolidation – beware of using anything high in fat in the first week.

I adore Hollandaise sauce. For years I didn't eat it because I, like so many people, was afraid of the fat it contains. This recipe is easy to make, low in carbs and tastes great over cooked spinach or asparagus. Use it as a dipping sauce for artichokes as well.

WHAT YOU NEED
100g butter
4 egg yolks
juice of 1 lemon
Himalayan or Malvern salt, to taste
freshly ground black pepper, to taste
1 teaspoon Dijon mustard (optional)
sprinkling of Mexican chilli powder (optional)

HERE'S HOW
Melt one third of the butter in a basin set over a pan of simmering water (a bain-marie), then remove from the heat. Beat the egg yolks in a bowl, using either a hand-held electric beater or a whisk. Very slowly add the melted butter to the egg yolks, continuing to mix all the time. Pour this mixture back into the bain-marie and put back over simmering water. Gradually add the rest of the butter, little by little, all the while continuing to whisk. Once the butter is completely melted and integrated with the sauce, remove it from the heat, stir in the lemon juice, salt, pepper and other ingredients.

Easy Mayonnaise
makes about 300ml
vegetarian

Good for Weeks 2–6 of Consolidation – beware of using anything high in fat in the first week.

Mayonnaise is not as difficult to make as everybody seems to believe, particularly since the advent of high-speed blenders and food processors. It does take a little bit of patience and a little bit of practice. If by any chance you don't succeed with your first emulsion, simply wash out and carefully dry your blender or food processor then use the 'unemulsified emulsion' to drop back, drop by drop, into a new supply of egg yolks as though it were oil itself. Naturally you will have to add a bit more seasoning, as you'll end up with a bit more mayonnaise.

This mayonnaise is made with extra-virgin olive oil, but you have the option of substituting flaxseed oil for part of the olive oil. You can do all sorts of wonderful things to it, like add nuts, garlic, herbs and mustards. Commercial mayonnaise – the kind you buy in jars in the supermarket – is something you want to avoid. It is full of trans-fatty acids and made from the cheapest, nastiest forms of hydrogenated junk fats. Mayonnaise you make yourself will keep for 4–5 days in the coolest part of the refrigerator. Here's my basic recipe, plus some suggestions on how to vary it.

WHAT YOU NEED
2 large egg yolks
275ml extra-virgin olive oil
2 tablespoons apple cider vinegar
2 tablespoons lemon juice
1/2 teaspoon dry mustard
Himalayan or Malvern salt, to taste
freshly ground black pepper, to taste

HERE'S HOW

Put the egg yolks in a blender or food processor and begin to blend on a low setting. Very, very gradually add the oil – literally drop by drop as the blender is running until you see an emulsion starting to happen. When this begins you will no longer be seeing liquid swirling round and round, but something thicker, with the consistency of a light face cream. Continue slowly adding oil to the mixture in a thin stream, all the while keeping the blender setting on low, until you have added half the oil. Then put in the vinegar, lemon juice, mustard, salt and pepper, all the while continuing to blend. Finally, slowly add the remaining oil. Taste and adjust seasoning.

Go-for-Garlic Mayonnaise

Add 2–4 crushed cloves of garlic when you are adding the lemon juice for an intense garlicky mayonnaise.

Orange Zest

Leave out the mustard when making mayonnaise, but instead add 2 teaspoons grated orange zest, a tablespoon fresh orange juice and 2 tablespoons finely chopped fresh mint leaves to 240ml mayonnaise.

Curried Mayonnaise

To 120ml of your home-made mayonnaise add 1 teaspoon mild to medium curry powder and a teaspoon of finely grated fresh ginger.

Tofu Mayonnaise Lite
vegan

This mayonnaise, instead of being made with oil, is made with tofu. You can use it for salads and dips as well as sauces to go on cooked vegetables. It's easy to make and light as air to eat. Like conventional mayonnaise, you can vary this recipe by adding garlic, cajun seasoning (see page 163), mustard or fresh herbs to give a totally different flavour.

WHAT YOU NEED

450g soft tofu, drained

50g granular lecithin

3 tablespoons lemon juice

small pinch of stevia (optional)

1 teaspoon Marigold Swiss Vegetable Bouillon or Rapunzel Organic
   Vegetable Bouillon powder

50ml extra-virgin olive oil

1 teaspoon finely grated lemon zest

Himalayan or Malvern salt, to taste

freshly ground black pepper, to taste

HERE'S HOW

Put the tofu into a blender and add the lecithin granules, lemon juice, stevia and bouillon powder, as well as half the oil. Blend well until thoroughly mixed. Now slowly, drop by drop, add the remaining oil and blend again for 2–4 minutes until the mixture grows thick and creamy. Finally stir in the lemon zest and season with salt and pepper. This mixture will keep in the refrigerator for 5–6 days.

Avocado Delight
vegan

Good for all six weeks of Consolidation.

This is a superb dip or dressing, and very rich indeed. Excellent on a sprout salad or as a dip for crudités.

WHAT YOU NEED
1 avocado, peeled and stoned
juice of 1 lemon
juice of 1/2 orange
1 small onion, finely chopped
1 clove garlic, finely chopped
handful of fresh herbs (mint, parsley or basil)
Himalayan or Malvern salt, to taste
freshly ground black pepper, to taste

HERE'S HOW
Blend all the ingredients in a food processor or blender and serve. This dressing will not keep for more than one day in the fridge.

DELICIOUS GRAIN-FREE DISHES

Kasha
serves 4
vegan

Good for Weeks 4–6 of Consolidation.

Since kasha is not a grain but a seed, it almost never triggers food sensitivities. It has been a favourite for me ever since a Russian lover taught me how to make this traditional dish. It makes a wonderful breakfast – especially to share in bed on a Sunday morning.

WHAT YOU NEED

450g buckwheat groats

1 litre or more stock or water with 2 teaspoons Marigold Swiss
   Vegetable Bouillon or Rapunzel Organic Vegetable Bouillon powder

1 clove garlic, crushed

1/2 handful of chopped fresh mixed herbs

HERE'S HOW

Place the buckwheat in a heavy-bottomed pan and roast it dry over medium heat, stirring all the while with a wooden spoon. As it begins to darken, pour hot stock over it and add the garlic and 1 teaspoon of the herbs. Cover and simmer very slowly for about 15–20 minutes until all the liquid has been absorbed. Serve sprinkled with the remaining herbs.

Wild Rice

serves 4–6

Good for Weeks 4–6 of Consolidation.

My recipe uses a product native to the North–Central United States – wild rice. Wild rice is not actually a rice – it is a type of wild grass. It used to be a staple in the diet of Native Americans. It has a marvellous crunchy texture and almost never causes food sensitivities in people.

WHAT YOU NEED

340g uncooked wild rice, washed

1 litre water

1 teaspoon Himalayan or Malvern salt

4 slices bacon, diced

60g butter

1 small onion, chopped

1/2 cup celery, sliced

1/2 cup fresh mushrooms, sliced

1/4 teaspoon pepper

120g salted cashews (optional)

HERE'S HOW

Place wild rice, water and salt in a heavy saucepan. Bring to the boil, reduce to a simmer and cook for 45 minutes or until tender. Uncover and fluff with a fork. Simmer for a further 5 minutes, then drain. While the rice is cooking, fry the bacon until crisp. Drain on paper towels. In a frying pan, melt the butter and sauté the onion, celery and mushrooms until tender. Add the wild rice, season with salt and pepper, and heat through. Just before serving, top with the cashews and bacon pieces.

PROTEIN DISHES

Hand-made Sausages
serves 4

Good for all six weeks of Consolidation.

I adore sausages. But the sausages that you buy are full of all sorts of artificial flavouring, colourings and preservatives, not to mention cereal-based carbohydrate 'stuffers' which you want to avoid. This is an old-fashioned patty sausage which you can vary, depending upon your taste and what herbs and meats you have available. You can make it with pork, venison, chicken, lamb, beef or wild boar. I mix the ingredients together the night before, then put them in the fridge to chill and absorb all the flavours. Use within three days of preparing.

WHAT YOU NEED

350g lean minced pork, chicken, lamb, beef, venison or wild boar
1 teaspoon Himalayan or Malvern salt, to taste
2 tablespoons gram flour (besan/chickpea flour)
4 cloves garlic (optional)
2 tablespoons chopped fresh parsley, coriander or sage
1/2 large onion, finely chopped

HERE'S HOW

Combine all the ingredients in a big mixing bowl and mix thoroughly with your hands. Refrigerate until well chilled, then separate into four patties and cook in an oiled skillet until crunchy on the surface and cooked through.

Chicken Curry

serves 4

Good for all six weeks of Consolidation.

Curry is a dream-to-make low carb. It is creamy, thick, full of spices, with a rich fragrance and flavour. I often prepare it using leftover pieces of chicken, tossing them into a frying pan, mixing in all my sauce ingredients, then serving over a plate of lightly steamed broccoli or cauliflower florets.

Another way I make it – the really lazy way – is to cut a chicken in pieces and put it into a large cast-iron pot with a lid. I then toss in all the ingredients (except the coconut oil). Pop them into the oven with the lid on, and cook for about an hour at 200°C. Turn the chicken so that the sauce covers it and cook for another 15 minutes. This way you end up with curried chicken pieces you can enjoy any time you want for snacks or main courses.

Here is my recipe for a more conventionally made chicken curry.

WHAT YOU NEED

2 tablespoons coconut oil
3 tablespoons chives, chopped
6 cloves garlic, chopped
2 tablespoons green onions, chopped
1 good-sized piece fresh ginger, finely sliced
2 teaspoons mild or medium curry powder
pinch or two of cayenne pepper
pinch of turmeric

1 large chicken, skinned, boned and cut into bite-sized chunks
1 400ml can coconut milk
Himalayan or Malvern salt, to taste
freshly ground black pepper, to taste
handful of fresh parsley, chopped
chilli, to taste
parsley, to taste
stevia, to taste

HERE'S HOW
Melt the coconut oil in a heavy pot. Add the chives, garlic, onion and ginger and brown lightly. Toss in the curry powder and spices. Put in the chicken pieces and coat them with the sauce, allowing them to cook lightly for 2–3 minutes. Now cover and turn the heat down until the chicken pieces cook through, stirring every 5 minutes to make sure that nothing burns. Finally, pour on the coconut milk, add a little water if you need more juice, season with salt and pepper, bring to a simmer and cook gently for another 4 minutes. Season with chilli, parsley and stevia and serve.

Salmon Delight
serves 2

Good for all six weeks of Consolidation.

Salmon is a delightful fish with a unique, delicate flavour. I really love this lemony dish because it is so easy to prepare and so tasty. The marinade enhances the natural flavours of the fish and the spring onion gives zest.

WHAT YOU NEED
2 large spring onions, finely chopped
juice of 4 medium-sized lemons
Himalayan or Malvern salt, to taste

pepper, to taste
2 fillets salmon
1 dessertspoon coconut oil
zest of 1 lemon, 2 lemon wedges and parsley (for garnish)

HERE'S HOW
Put the spring onions in a mixing bowl. Add the lemon juice, salt and pepper and blend. Place the salmon fillets in the marinade, skin side up, and leave for 45 minutes. Turn the fillets over and leave for a further 15 minutes. Heat the coconut oil in a frying pan. Drain the fillets, place them in the pan and sauté until tender. Serve with lemon garnish.

HOT VEGETABLES

Try using cauliflower instead of potatoes to thicken your soups or sauces. Use gram flour (also called besan or chickpea flour) instead of wheat flour to thicken sauces. Try substituting the vegetables you are used to using – say potatoes or sweet potatoes – with low-carb ones. If you want to dredge your fish or chicken dishes in flour, again use some gram flour, or ground almonds or macadamias, before cooking. Enjoy dips with flaxseed crackers (see page 256), whole leaves of chicory, celery or sweet peppers cut into wedges, instead of ordinary crackers or toast. Instead of a flour crust, make a flan using a flaxseed or nut-and-flaxseed crust – great for supplying natural fibre. You can also do without a crust altogether by buttering your pan well and pouring the eggs directly into it.

Baked Asparagus
serves 4

Good for all six weeks of Consolidation.

Not only does asparagus appear in early spring with a very short growing season – which makes it seem ultra-desirable – but it is also a powerfully healing vegetable. It has long been used in Ayurvedic medicine as a remedy against indigestion. You can cut asparagus into pieces and pop them into the steamer – the heavier ends first and the little tips afterwards. I like to serve steamed or baked asparagus with wedges of lemon and shaved Parmesan, plus a little garlic salt and pepper. You can also use a pesto or mayonnaise (see pages 257 and 259–61) and serve it hot or cold.

WHAT YOU NEED
3 dozen asparagus spears, trimmed and peeled if necessary
2–3 tablespoons melted butter or olive oil
Himalayan or Malvern salt, to taste
coarsely ground pepper, to taste
1 lemon, divided into 6 wedges

HERE'S HOW
Place the asparagus side by side in a rectangular baking dish and drizzle with butter or olive oil. Season with salt and pepper. Cover with a lid or with foil, then bake at 225°C for 20–30 minutes, depending upon the thickness of the asparagus – that is, until the spears are browned and tender. Add a little extra melted butter and serve with a wedge of lemon on each plate. Can be enjoyed warm or cold.

Chargrilled Sweet Peppers
serves 4

Good for Weeks 2–6 of Consolidation.

Another great way of cooking vegetables is to chargrill them with a little olive oil. They make a good vegetable accompaniment to a main course. Or you can eat them, as I like to, as a meal on their own, hot or cold, when you're not terribly hungry. Many vegetables lend themselves to chargrilling. Although this recipe is for sweet peppers, you can use it with red onions, tomatoes, courgettes, aubergines, fennel, celery, cauliflower and broccoli. Even Brussels sprouts, which are by no means my favourite vegetable, come out well when chargrilled.

I serve chargrilled vegetables just as they come, marinated in the sauce that I use to baste them. Sometimes I squeeze extra lemon juice over them.

WHAT YOU NEED
8 sweet peppers, red, yellow or green
1 red onion, chopped
4 cloves garlic, finely sliced

For the marinade
8 tablespoons olive oil
1/2 teaspoon tamari
zest and juice of 1 lime (use lemon if you can't find lime)
2 cloves garlic, finely chopped
2 teaspoons bright red peppercorns, ground in a mortar and pestle
2 tablespoons shallots, finely chopped

For the garnish
small handful of finely chopped fresh herbs – tarragon, basil,
   coriander, flat-leaved parsley or fennel

HERE'S HOW

Combine the ingredients for the marinade and mix well. Pour into a flat pan. Cut the sweet peppers in half, remove the seeds and add to the marinade. Allow them to sit for between 15 minutes and 2–3 hours, turning occasionally so that they soak up the marinade. Now you're ready to cook – either on a cast-iron chargrill pan, a teppenyaki grill (my favourite method), underneath the grill of your oven or atop the barbecue. Your grilling surface should be extremely hot. Check this by splashing it with a bit of water: the water drops should jump high, then disappear altogether. Place the sweet peppers, red onion and garlic cloves on your grill or pan, backside to the heat first, and cook until brown, turning them over as necessary and brushing on more of the marinade as you go. Turn them and finish off on the open side, filling the centre of the sweet peppers with more of the marinade. Just before serving, squeeze on some lemon juice and sprinkle with fresh herbs. Alternatively, serve them in a little pile on each dish so that people can sprinkle them with herbs if they wish. Add freshly ground red peppercorns and serve with ribbons of lemon skin around the vegetables on each plate.

JUST DESSERTS

What's your favourite? Chocolate mousse? Lemon Cream Pie? On Consolidation you can enjoy them all. None of my recipes contains sugar or artificial sweeteners such as aspartame or saccharin. Instead, they make use of stevia. Stevia extracts – the white stevia or the liquid form – work best in most desserts, as both dried and fresh leaves tend to turn things green. (I have yet to be seduced by the idea of a green meringue!)

Almond Macaroons
makes 18

Good for all six weeks of Consolidation, but test for sensitivity to eggs and nuts first.

This is my version of the delicious amaretti biscuits from Italy which simply melt in your mouth. They are easy to make, have only 1.5g of carbohydrate per biscuit and are delicious with tea or at the end of a meal.

WHAT YOU NEED
50g finely ground almonds (best done in a coffee grinder)
50g unsweetened, finely shredded desiccated coconut
1 teaspoon vanilla essence (the *real* thing – no sugar, preferably
   organic)
1 tablespoon almond-flavoured liqueur or almond essence (optional)
stevia, to taste
pinch of Himalayan or Malvern salt, to taste
2 free-range or organic egg whites
1 tablespoon coconut oil or butter, for greasing the baking sheet

HERE'S HOW
Preheat the oven to 145°C. Mix the ground almonds together with the coconut, vanilla, almond liqueur and salt, then set aside. Beat the egg whites in a separate bowl. Fold in the other ingredients and mix gently with your fingers. Roll the mixture into balls the size of large marbles and place on a greased baking sheet. Bake for 20–25 minutes or until golden brown yet still soft inside.

Easygoing Pie Crust
vegan

Good for all six weeks of Consolidation, but test for sensitivity to nuts first, and always use them sparingly.

This pie crust, which is made from fresh almonds and flaxseeds, is healthfully rich in the omega-3 and omega-6 fatty acids. I use it for just about everything, from a frozen raspberry pie to a cheesecake. I like to grind up my flaxseeds in a coffee grinder. I do the same with the almonds. I find that coffee grinders reduce things to a beautiful powder that you can easily manipulate into whatever you want.

WHAT YOU NEED
60g flaxseeds, ground to a fine powder
1 teaspoon fresh lemon juice
2–4 tablespoons iced water
stevia, to taste
pinch of salt
180g almonds, ground to a fine powder
1 1/2 tablespoons coconut oil, melted

HERE'S HOW
Soak the ground flaxseeds in the lemon juice and a couple of teaspoons of iced water for 20 minutes. Mix together with a fork and put aside. In another bowl mix together the stevia and salt with the almonds and the melted coconut oil. Now combine the seed and nut mixtures, stirring with your fingers until mixed thoroughly. Pour into a 22cm flan dish and, using your fingers, press the mixture into the pan all along the bottom and the sides. Prick with a knife or fork and bake at 160°C for 15 minutes. Allow to cool, then you are ready to fill.

Lemon Cream Pie
serves 8

Good for all six weeks of Consolidation, but test for sensitivity to sour cream, cream and cottage cheese first.

This is one of the fillings that I use for pies. It's creamy and yummy. You can make similar recipes using pumpkin, strawberries or rhubarb. You can even make chocolate cream pies and strawberry cream pies – all it takes is a little imagination.

WHAT YOU NEED

120ml fresh lemon juice
125g unflavoured gelatin
stevia, to taste
450g cottage cheese
240ml sour cream
1 teaspoon finely grated lemon zest
200ml double cream, whipped
60g fresh raspberries, blackberries, blueberries or strawberries,
    crushed and sweetened with a little stevia

HERE'S HOW

Heat half the lemon juice gently in a saucepan, sprinkling the gelatin into it and stirring over a low heat until dissolved. Mix the stevia together with the cottage cheese, blending in the sour cream, the remainder of the lemon juice and the lemon zest. Now mix in the lemon gelatin mixture and blend well. Cool in a refrigerator until the mixture has thickened but not set completely. Fold in the whipped cream. Spoon the filling into a pie crust and chill for several hours. Serve with the crushed berries as a topping.

New Beginnings

THERE IS NO GREATER JOY than feeling fully alive – living in the moment the way a child does, protected from the ravages of premature ageing and degeneration. You can call on high levels of energy when you need them, surrender to blissful relaxation when you choose to and live out even more of your innate capacity for joy and creativity. On a physical/energetic level, what all this depends on is the condition of the *living matrix*.

Your Living Matrix

In the early 1990s a revolutionary paradigm was created, bringing with it a deeper understanding of how living systems function in health and disease. Leading-edge researchers and scientists realized that it is both misleading and inaccurate to treat the body as little more than a collection of organs, muscles, bones and chemicals, as most modern medicine continues to do. More accurately, they concluded, your body is a fluid, dynamic, continuous webwork of energy, physical substance and light – a living matrix. This unique matrix behaves like a multi-dimensional, molecular continuum which is not only physical but energetic. It integrates all the body's parts and activities. It even has semi-conductor properties.

All the regulatory processes on which health depends take place within the living matrix. When we nourish our own living matrix well on every level it rewards us with radiant vitality and lasting leanness. New England scientist Dr James L. Oschman, author of *Energy Medicine – The Scientific Basis*, is an articulate and exacting researcher into the nature of the living matrix, how it works and what improves its functioning. He has even developed ways of measuring beneficial effects on the matrix from such diverse practices as yoga, Chinese qigong, laying on of hands, and Reiki healing. When the matrix functions with a high degree of energetic order, your body is vital and resistant to degeneration. It also heals easily.

Stories the Genes Can Tell

There are many ways to nourish your living matrix – through the foods you eat, the energetic fields to which you do and don't allow yourself to be exposed, an ongoing awareness of what your body is asking from you, and a willingness to listen and act upon the messages it sends. We will be exploring some of these in the next section, 'The Transformation'. But before we do, let's take one more look at the role genes have to play in all this and examine some exciting discoveries about *genetic expression*, which will change for ever any belief you may still hold that we are all prisoners to the genes we have inherited from our family.

Discoveries from the Human Genome Project vie in importance with Darwin's discoveries about evolution a century before. The Human Genome Project was focused on analysing the almost six billion pieces of DNA that make up our genes. The volume of information about health and disease patterns hidden within them is breathtaking and continues to emerge. Even twenty-five years ago the idea that disease patterns might be identified through our genes looked like science fiction. Now it is common knowledge.

To the uninformed, the idea that our health, biological age and death are written in our genes sounds depressing – akin to some mean-minded clairvoyant predicting that our future is something we are powerless to change. This is simply untrue.

Transformation through expression

Far more exciting than the discovery that specific genes can make us either susceptible or resistant to specific illnesses is a lesser-known, yet far more powerful, revelation that has also emerged from the Human Genome Project. While it is true that our genes define our 'risk' of early ageing, degeneration and obesity, whether or not this 'risk' becomes a 'fact' depends far less on our genetic inheritance than on how we choose to live our lives. The truth is this: it is not the genes that give rise to disease and degeneration in a living body. It is the way our genes are *expressed*.

Let me explain. There are many possible versions of you tucked away in your genes and chromosomes. Which version gets expressed – which of your genetic potentials become manifest as reality in your life – depends more on the way you live than on any gene risk factors. The simple changes you have brought about with the help of Cura Romana – changes in the way you eat, use your body, handle stress and orientate yourself spiritually and creatively – can set you on the road to excellent genetic expression in your life, provided you continue to honour your body, stay conscious of its needs and do your best to provide them as the years pass. But wait – there's better news. Even if signs of degeneration have already appeared, it is often possible to reverse them – rejuvenating your body and mind in medically measurable ways.

Back in time – a final glance

'Gene expression' is the scientific term for how you manage genetic inheritance in your day-to-day life. Do your genes express themselves by creating massive vitality for you? Clarity of mind? Creativity? Freedom from illness? Or do they express themselves in negative ways by creating obesity, sagging skin and spirit, early ageing and degeneration? The quality of our genetic expression depends to an enormous degree on how well we take care of the living matrix, and also on how well we honour our general genetic inheritance, refined over two million years. This is one of the reasons that every now and then it can be useful to check back with the chart below. It may remind you of things you have forgotten – things we all forget, living the busy lives we do.

Palaeolithic Diet	Modern Western Diet
No cereal or grain-based carbohydrates (they didn't exist). No sugars. No genetically modified foods.	75% of our foods made from cereal- and grain-based carbohydrates and/or sugars, including fructose – often in the form of corn syrup.
Drinks consisted of water and mother's milk. No milk products from animals.	Drinks consist of coffee, alcohol, cow's-milk beverages, sports drinks, sodas and diet sodas, replete with dangerous artificial sweeteners, chemicals and flavourings.
More than 200 kinds of raw fruits and vegetables. Starchy vegetables, such as modern potatoes, grains and our contemporary rice, did not exist.	On average we consume fewer than 20 different foods, very few fresh raw vegetables and large quantities of manufactured foods for which our body has no genetic reference.
60–90% of calories consumed came in the form of proteins – small and large game animals, eggs, birds, fish, shellfish, reptiles and insects.	80% of the calories we consume each day come from refined sugars, dairy products, cereals and grains, sugars and starchy vegetables.
Ratio of omega-6 fats to omega-3 fats consumed was between 1:1 and 3:1, since their animals were replete with essential fatty acids as well as some saturated fats. The best balance is 2:1 or 3:1 omega 6 and omega 3, which our hunter-gatherer ancestors got.	Ratio of omega-6 fats to omega-3 fats consumed is now 22:1. Our domesticated animals contain virtually no essential fatty acids as they too are fed on grains. Our convenience foods, such as golden oils and margarines, are full of distorted fat molecules such as trans-fatty acids, anathema to the health of the body.

The Road Ahead

Simeons insisted that, after completing Cura Romana, every one of his former patients continue to weigh naked on rising each day. This was not an attempt to make them fearful that they might regain weight lost. Daily weighing is an important and useful indicator that the diencephalic reset for appetite and weight control that took place during Cura Romana continues to function as it is meant to. This way your body will not be led to believe that you are asking it to revert to its former ways of functioning, which had been causing weight gain in the past. Daily weighing is also a useful way of keeping in touch with your body. It is easy for any of us to get so involved in the outside of our lives that we forget how essential it is to honour and nourish our living matrix.

> **Simeons says:** *Many patients think that this is unnecessary and that they can judge any increase from the fit of their clothes. Some do not carry their scale with them on a journey as it is cumbersome and takes a big bite out of their luggage-allowance when flying. This is a disastrous mistake, because after a course of hCG as much as 10 lbs. can be regained without any noticeable change in the fit of the clothes. The reason for this is that after treatment newly acquired fat is at first evenly distributed and does not show the former preference for certain parts of the body.*

Manoeuvring in the World

The question I am most often asked at the end of Consolidation is how to continue to give your body what it wants and needs when you have to travel, to entertain, to eat meals in restaurants frequently. Navigating when you're away from home is not as difficult as you might imagine. There are a few tricks that can be really helpful for negotiating the complex world of foods and snacks once you walk out of the front door.

Simple is best

Good restaurants can be easy away-from-home eating solutions provided they let you specify what you want. The best restaurants are invariably the easiest. They cook their food to order, in contrast to fast-food places where foods are pre-packaged and come whatever way they happen to be served. In a restaurant where foods are cooked to order, you can pretty much write your own ticket. You might have green beans or asparagus with a spinach side salad to go with sea bass steamed or grilled in butter and garlic, instead of served (as it states on the menu) smothered in what seems to you a questionable sauce. The toughest restaurants, apart from fast-food chains, are those that are known as 'health-food restaurants'. The name can be deceiving. Their dishes can be chock full of flour, honey and raw sugar. If you get stuck in one of these, it's best to go for a salad and see if they have some tofu you can eat with it, or get them to make you a sugar-free smoothie from raw greens and micro-filtered whey.

Japanese is easy

I love Japanese restaurants, first because the food is so good in general, and second because they are some of the easiest places in the world to get simple foods. Order sashimi plus a beautiful Japanese sprout salad with umeboshi vinegar. But make sure the raw fish is fresh. Most of the fish the Japanese serve are rich in precious omega-3 fatty acids. If you have any doubts about the fish being served in a restaurant, never eat it raw – there can always be a risk of parasite contamination. This makes me careful about the Japanese restaurants I choose, particularly when I'm in the northern hemisphere. In the southern hemisphere, the fish is often so fresh that I don't need to worry about it. Teppenyaki is an ideal dish anywhere. So is teriyaki chicken, or beef and salad (always ask for sauces to be made without any sugar), seaweed broth, miso soup and tofu. Stay away from tempura, since it is battered then fried in oils, which you are usually better off without.

Mexican is hot

Mexican food is a bit of a hotch-potch. There are some workable ways to go, however. Order a tostada or taco salad. Unless you know your body handles wheat or corn well, don't eat the shell beneath. Fajitas work well too, because you can easily avoid the tortillas that come on the side. Grilled fish, beef, pork medallions, chicken, as well as shredded beef, chicken or pork are great served with a mixed salad. Mexican restaurants usually have a good selection of fish served Veracruz style with tomatoes, sweet peppers and onions. I adore red snapper prepared this way. Ask for a salsa or guacamole made with olive oil on the side (much guacamole gets made with cheap vegetable oils). Gazpacho is a great soup for starters.

The French connection

French restaurants are almost always easy. You can always get a gorgeous salad (ask for extra-large), as well as grilled or poached fish, any kind of roasted game or meat. Make sure that none of the sauces that come with your main course is made from flour (fewer and fewer are these days).

When in Rome

Italian restaurants are a cinch – if you avoid the breads and pasta. I go for a grilled calamari (squid) salad to start, or an antipasto plate followed by grilled chicken breast, grilled fish or unbreaded veal, and one of those wonderful Italian salads brimming with herbs, radicchio and rocket, smothered in extra-virgin olive oil and spiked with fat Italian olives. It makes me hungry just to think about it.

Great Greek food

Souvlaki – skewered lamb, beef, chicken or shrimp kebabs with vegetables – works beautifully. What you will probably want to avoid are the pastries, breads and pastas used in Middle Eastern and Greek cooking. Their salads are wonderful, particularly those full of feta cheese with olive oil and red wine vinegar dressing. Even the yogurt tzatziki sauce, which they sometimes pour on top, is delicious.

In the air

Airlines are still a hassle. Despite dozens of years of preparing 'special meals', including kosher, vegetarian, vegan and the like, you would think that none of the catering directors of any of the airlines has ever heard of high-raw, low-grain eating. I travel a lot. Many of my travels are long-haul flights, some of which take more than 24 hours, so I try to plan this part of my life pretty carefully.

Some of the food on airlines, of course, you can eat. The simpler it is the better. Things like steamed fish and cheese are usually manageable. If you order a 'kosher meal' in advance, you are less likely to get some silly sauce poured over your fish or meat, but they are still going to provide you with ghastly rolls and yucky desserts. Often you can explain to the cabin crew (if you are not sitting in business or first class) that you are on a special diet and unfortunately the airline was not able to fulfil your needs. Then ask them if it is possible to gather together some fish, meat, salads and other relatively simple foods from the first-class menu for you. Most flight attendants are willing to do this.

Instant nourishment

When I'm travelling or simply out for the day, I often carry a plastic shaker with me, as well as a couple of little plastic bags, into which I put a good dose of micro-filtered whey protein plus a good powdered green supplement. Then all I have to do is pour clean water into the shaker, add my protein/green powder mix, shake it up and drink it. I carry this special back-up with me often, even to meetings, so that I am never forced to eat food that I don't want. Whatever else happens, I know at the very least that micro-filtered whey protein plus green will carry me through to my next decent meal.

Neo-Apple Days

Travelling on planes or trains can be a perfect time to do a variation on Simeons' Apple Day theme, with no restrictions on how many apples you eat and drinking as much clean water as you can. Not only is lots of liquid a good antidote to the dehydrating effects of cabin air, but this helps relieve jet lag. On the other hand, what slows down recovery from jet lag is eating meals at strange times. On west–east transatlantic flights, for example, you might be served breakfast at 4 a.m. or midnight 'body time'. Eating only apples and drinking lots of water or herbal teas helps you avoid this problem and arrive at your destination feeling lighter and livelier, instead of tired with indigestion. Make the first meal at your destination (be it breakfast, lunch or dinner) a light fruit or vegetable salad with good lean protein if you feel hungry.

Facing Your Future

People at the further reaches of human health don't look towards the future with fears of getting old and falling prey to degenerative conditions. They live in anticipation that the best is yet to come. They have discovered that, no matter what their age, they are capable of moving towards an even more positive state of health and fulfilment as the years pass. They are no longer ruled by outdated notions of ageing which teach that, as we get older, illness becomes a 'natural' part of life. They know differently.

One of the most important gifts from Cura Romana – another thing that separates it from weightloss diets – is the way it empowers the living matrix, helping to restore order to body and mind. This encourages a myriad other health benefits that people regularly experience on the programme. The discoveries you have made for yourself in Consolidation about foods which support the vitality of your living matrix, as well as those which undermine its health and vitality, are an excellent foundation on which to build an even more positive genetic expression that will keep you thriving year after year.

PART FOUR

THE
TRANSFORMATION

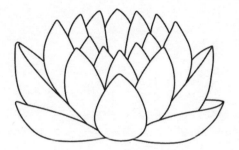

Journey to the Core

WITHIN EACH ONE of us there is a core of authentic power, creativity and joy. Gently, in silence, it waits for us to discover it, call it forth and set it free.

When I speak of the core, I mean that part of you which encompasses your essence – makes you different from each and every person who has ever lived. Far deeper than personality, your core is home to your essential being – the truth of who you are. The more we live from our core, the more authentic and rewarding our life becomes. Learn to live this way and you will be able to access universal life-energy and direct it towards whatever ends you choose.

> 'I discovered a lightness and a new sense of self. This program brought me so much more than I bargained for. It taught me how to trust, to listen to my body and just let go – to free-fall knowing I would safely land on my feet. All this and the weightloss was easy – what joy!'
> *Frances in the United States shed 20 pounds*

Despite Cura Romana's skills in helping people restore natural size, shape and weight to their bodies and improve their health, many men and women on the programme report that its greatest gift is the way it appears to help them discover who, in truth, they are and learn to live more of their lives from their essential being.

> 'The programme cleared away years of unwanted rubbish on a spiritual level which had been holding me back from living an authentic life – just being me and feeling good about it.'
> *Mary in England shed 12 pounds*

Spiritual Dimensions

Twenty years ago, when I was introduced to Cura Romana, I would never have dreamed that such a thing were possible. Now, after three years of working with people on the homeopathic programme we have developed, I am certain that something very special is going on – something that was not part of the original Protocol that relied on injectable hCG. Almost daily I receive reports from participants who speak of enriched spiritual experiences, some of which they consider life-changing.

> 'I felt that something important was taking place within the first week. My way of perceiving myself was different and I started to be more aware of what was going on in my body. My spiritual life became increasingly important; I started to realize that I was going through an inner transformation too.'
> *Myriam in France shed 37.5 pounds*

Like the proverbial iceberg, most of us live our lives with the lion's share of our potential for freedom, joy, bliss and creativity submerged beneath a sea of unknowing. We go about our day-to-day lives driven by unconscious assumptions about what is and what is not possible for us. Frequently we find ourselves swamped with anxieties, worries, depression or confusion.

> 'All the depression has gone and with it all the medication I took for 15 years. I am light and clear. A strange but wonderful emptiness of the old self has created the space for my true being to thrive.'
> *Karen in Scotland shed 17.5 pounds*

Yet, beneath the illusions, traumas, joys and chaos of the twenty-first century, our core of being carries only one intention: that each of us lives our life authentically, expressing as fully as possible our creativity, love, power and magnificence as we walk the earth.

This realization comes to many on the programme. Why this should be happening, I am still unsure. But when I became aware that something remarkable was taking place, this spurred me to work with John Morgan to devise a formula that would not only encompass the four homeopathic potencies of hCG directed entirely at fat-burning, but would also have a new, gentle potency added to support potentials for spiritual and emotional growth at the same time.

> 'Cura Romana is not yet another diet and weightloss programme. It is a passage through which our dreams, hopes and desires can become manifest – for a healthier, more authentic way of living by connecting with our inner core. It is a process of transformation – a priceless gift.'
> *Samina in England shed 12 pounds*

Fully Alive

To be fully alive we must be who we are, for who we are is far more interesting, vital and attractive than anything or anyone we might aspire to be. This fact is, sadly, often forgotten. Cura Romana is a time in which, thanks to the diencephalic changes taking place via the autonomic nervous system to body, brain and hormones, we are offered the finest opportunity that I have yet come across to connect with the true nature of our own being, if we choose to take it.

> **Simeons says:** *Buried deep down in the massive human brain there is a part which we have in common with all vertebrate animals, the so-called diencephalon. It is a very primitive part of the brain and has in man been almost smothered by the huge masses of nervous tissue with which we think, reason and voluntarily move our body. The diencephalon is the part from which the central nervous system controls all the automatic animal functions of the body, such as breathing, the heart beat, digestion, sleep, sex, the urinary system, the autonomous or vegetative nervous system and via the pituitary the whole interplay of the endocrine glands.*

It seems evident that such inner transformations begin as physiological and functional alterations in diencephalic functioning. Yet why they appear to happen so easily on the homeopathic version of the Protocol as opposed to the injectable one I do not yet understand. Has it to do with the energetic nature of the homeopathic acting upon not only the physicality of this complex regulatory system but also on subtle aspects of the living matrix which have not yet been charted? These are a few of the questions I continue to ask myself.

In his book *Man's Presumptuous Brain*, Simeons explores at length the conflicts that take place in civilized man between the primitive diencephalon and the highly developed cerebral cortex – conflicts which often result in illness. Is it possible that Cura Romana helps create more balance between our cool, rational conscious mind and our primitive, instinctual animal nature, thereby creating greater harmony between our bodies and our minds? After all, the body is the medium through which our lives unfold – a reality that we too often ignore. We live in a strange culture which pays far too little attention to the importance of connecting with the essential being – soul, if you like – thereby developing the potentials we humans have for expanded consciousness and welcoming higher levels of insight and bliss into our lives.

> 'Cura Romana has completely transformed my life. I wake up every morning energized and blissful. I am more aware of everything and everyone around me and, most important of all, I am more aware of my own needs and of myself.'
> *Mirjana in England shed 19.8 pounds*

Four-letter Word

The word 'soul' is often demeaned or dismissed, in no small part because of its association with – and exploitation by – organized religion. In truth the word 'soul' is far older than organized religion. It comes from Old English, Old Frisian, and back and back beyond that. 'Soul' means the essential part or fundamental nature of anything – its animating force – the seat of personality, intellect, will and emotion, the inspiring spirit that both guides us and causes movement.

Each human soul carries a powerful intention to realize its unique nature as fully as possible. And, like any living thing, it needs tending in order to blossom. The soul never forces itself into conscious awareness. Instead, it whispers to each of us, offering information we need to know if we are to become fulfilled and fully alive. It is our job to listen to its whispers. When we cannot hear them or do not heed them, we risk becoming fodder for any who would exploit our uncertainties by telling us that if only we change, become more reasonable, thinner, better educated, more tractable, buy the latest expensive car, then everything will be all right with our lives. We will fit in, we will belong.

Healthy young children often have a strong bridge between their essential self and their outer personality. It is second nature to them. They respond to the world directly, they speak their mind. They live each moment to the hilt, moving from one activity to another. But when they grow up – when *we* grow up – we take on too many assumptions, false ideas and other people's directives, so we weaken and lose track of this connection. This happens to all of us to one degree or another. Sometimes we even forget who we are, let alone how to live more of our lives from our authentic being.

> 'For the first time in my life I know that the strength and power to live my life to the full lies within me, thanks to Cura Romana. Today I saw myself standing on a cliff top with the wind blowing in my face as the world was opening up to me. I feel like the wind itself – strong and free!'
> *Vicki in New Zealand shed 27.5 pounds*

Everything You Need Is Within

An important part of reconnecting with the core is a willingness to leave behind any notion you still carry that what you need or long for has to come from outside yourself. In truth, everything we need for our own freedom and fulfilment we already have inside. It simply needs to be discovered, called forth and set free.

> 'For the first time ever, I feel that the next phase of my life will be really exciting and full of growth and more new experiences. Now I know I have the power to make it that way.'
> *Edward in Canada shed 32.7 pounds*

When I finally came to terms with how profound the emotional and spiritual changes can be for many on Cura Romana, I began to gather tools, techniques and information which I and those I have worked with have found to be useful in helping us reconnect with our core. I offered them to those I have been mentoring as a way of supporting spiritual processes which they told me had been initiated or intensified by the programme. You will find many of these simple processes in the chapters that follow. They are interesting, consciousness-expanding and fun to do. Try them out, use those that appeal to you and forget the rest. You might be surprised what a powerful role practising them regularly can play in reweaving that bridge between your inner and your outer life.

Expand Consciousness

When we are in our ordinary state of awareness, we often see the world and ourselves as though through a veil. We make use of only a very small part of our capacity for creativity, passion, joy and intuition. Once we begin to forge deeper connections with our core, we gain access to levels of awareness, experience and insight believed to be available only to artists and mystics, and gain even greater access to our authentic selves. The best way to explain what I mean is to show you. Try this as a first step.

The inner reaches

Here is a simple yet powerful exercise in guided imagery – a blissful, restorative practice you can use to unwind when you feel you need it. But it is far more than that too. Practising it regularly – both during and after your Cura Romana Journey – will help to build a powerful, creative bridge between the essential self and the personality that directs our day-to-day life. A great many studies in recent years have shown that the shifts brought about through guided imagery not only alleviate stress, bring the body and mind into a state of balance, and activate our natural healing capacities, but they give us access to the vast, multi-sensory realms, rich in creativity, intuition, vision, spiritual experiences, meaning and values. They also give us access to equally vast inner realms replete with treasures from the soul.

You can record the words below on an MP3 player or tape, then listen to them (be sure to leave spaces of silence after each statement so that your imagination can run free). Or you can just sit quietly with the book in your lap. Read each bullet point, then close your eyes and see where it takes you before going on to the next point.

Practising the Inner Reaches once or twice a week – even more often if you like – you will become familiar with your very own sacred place of silence and natural beauty. This is a sanctuary of absolute safety and a place to which you can return, no matter where you are or in what circumstances you find yourself. Use it for healing, for renewing your physical and mental energy, for cleansing your body or your psyche and for tapping into creativity whenever you wish. Most important of all – use it as a tool to discover who you are at the deepest levels of your being and begin to sense the authentic freedom just waiting for you to live it as you do.

Here's how:
- Turn off the phone so you won't be disturbed for the next 10 minutes.
- Sit on a straight-backed chair, or on the floor if you prefer. Take three or four nice deep breaths through your nose,

letting the air escape gently through your mouth on the out breath.

- Close your eyes.
- Put your imagination into gear. Let your mind go back to some place in nature which you have seen and which you especially like. This is a real place, not somewhere from a dream or a story. It may be a place familiar to you, say at the end of your garden. Or it can be somewhere you have visited only once.
- When you have found the place you like, sit for a moment quietly remembering as much about it as you can.
- Forget any concerns you may have about your day-to-day life. Allow the wind to carry them high into the sky and far away. Just sit in your skin in your sacred place and breathe softly.
- Now see what happens when you activate your senses.
- What do you smell?
- How does the air feel against your skin?
- Sense the earth beneath your body. What is it like?
- What do you see?
- Are there any trees or fruits or flowers around you?
- What do you hear?
- Is there any water there? If so, can you hear it?
- Touch it?
- Drink some of it if you like.
- What does it feel like? Taste like?
- Are there stones nearby? If so, pick one up in your hand and feel the weight of it. Is it rough or smooth?
- What is the atmosphere like? Is the sun shining? Is there mist? Rain? Feel it on your body. Let it penetrate your clothes.
- Let yourself sink into the beauty that surrounds you. In a very real sense this beauty *is* you. All that you see in this special place is part of you and you are part of it.
- Are there any others there with you? Animals? People? Nature spirits? Helpers?

- Let yourself sense the energy of love that surrounds you. It is embedded within your very body by the beauty and the friendship that you take in.
- Simply *allow* the deepest levels of your being to speak to you – in words, in images, in sensations, in feelings. It doesn't matter. You may hear whispers about what delights you, about what you fear, about what you long for.
- When you are ready, give thanks for the friendship and the beauty around you and say goodbye for the moment to your inner sanctuary, knowing that you can return to it whenever you like.
- This place is yours and yours alone. You can come here to find the answer to a question, or for healing, clarity, renewal or refreshment.
- The more often you return, the richer the experience will become and the more valuable will be the gifts you bring back for yourself and others.
- Now, very gently, in your own time, open your eyes and come back into the room.

Bridge-building

Now take out your Cura Romana Journal and record what you have experienced in the Inner Reaches exercise. Describe it in words – where you went, what you saw, felt, tasted, sensed, who was there, what happened. If already you are beginning to hear gentle whispers from your soul, write down what this is like. Just let the words flow. Keep writing, without stopping or reading, until you have finished. Remember this is not an essay for school. There is no right or wrong way of doing this. If you prefer you can draw what you have seen. This does not have to be a literal drawing, that is of a tree, a flower, a rock; it can simply be colours swirled together to give the feeling of the place. What I like to do best is to use a combination of words and colours to record my perceptions and experiences. When using colour, the same guidelines apply as for the words – just let rip. You are not trying to be an 'artist' and there is no judgement involved. Let whatever comes on to the page happen. Recording what you experience in your journal – whatever that may be – is an effective way to rebuild that bridge between your authentic self and your day-to-day life.

The Courage to Be

To live at peace with ourselves, to ride the waves of our biological, spiritual and emotional energy with grace and confidence (and to make the best use of all three), three skills can be useful:

1 Awareness and a respect for the cyclic nature of energy and an appreciation of all its different qualities.

2 Knowing how to manage our energy when it needs managing – how to get down when we are stressed, how to heighten vitality when we feel low, and how to access stamina and sustained power when we need them for long-term efforts.

3 Cultivating the art of living from the core by welcoming the dissolution of any obstructions that may be interfering with full expression of our authenticity. For there, at the deepest centre of your being, at the source of all your hopes and dreams, a font of radiance unique to you alone is to be found. Tap into it and you access energies for health, joy and creativity of which most of us only dream.

> 'Without clearing the body and soul as Cura Romana does, we cannot open to our spirit-self. The program isn't an overnight fix but a complete life change at soul level.'
> *Jessie in the United States shed 18 pounds*

The more we connect with our essential being, the more radiance is ignited. Sooner or later, it begins to blaze forth in ways that enrich our own lives beyond measure, while blessing the lives of those around us at the same time.

STRIKE FOR
FREEDOM

THE EIGHTEENTH-CENTURY French philosopher Jean-Jacques Rousseau had a saying for which he is famous: 'Man is born free, yet everywhere he is in chains.' The essence of what he wrote is as true now as it was then. Each of us is born with a passion for freedom and an infinite capacity for realizing it. Then what keeps us from living out our freedom with enthusiasm, commitment and respect for ourselves? Of what are the chains that bind us made? How can we free ourselves from them? Most important of all, what kind of life awaits us when we do?

When Aaron and I began to work with our homeopathic Protocol, we would never have anticipated that the most commonly reported non-physical benefit felt by participants on completing the programme is an experience of expanded freedom. Each person describes this in his or her individual way. Some tell us that, often for the first time, a burden of conformity has been lifted away. 'I am lighter,' they say, 'not just in my body but in my being. I am free just to be me.' Others say that long-held limiting beliefs have 'lifted away'. Others claim that their lives and the world itself look different now –

'like everything is brand new'. So widespread are the reports we get about a greater sense of freedom that many of the materials you find in this section of the book have been chosen to support this mysterious expansive process and help you, if you wish, to a greater experience of freedom in your own life.

Freedom has always fascinated me. I love the smell of the word. I like its sense of possibility. I taste freedom when I listen to the music of Aaron Copland – music that could only have been written in a country that once had vast prairies and seemingly infinite wilderness. I feel it in my body when I run along cliffs in the rain. I rejoice in the sense of it that comes when, after hours of shifting dead words and sentences, something suddenly comes alive and beauty spills out all over the page.

Birthright

I sense that each of us longs for greater freedom. Rightly so. Freedom, like air and food and water, must be one of our human birthrights. Yet often we have little idea how to go about finding it. In their search for freedom, some end up sniffing cocaine or drinking cocktails. Others dance all weekend at a rave. A few turn to philosophy or look for it by reading self-help books or ancient sutras. Or maybe they head off to India or California to sit at the foot of a guru, hoping, somehow, he or she will hand it to them. All these things – from rum and cocaine to raves and yoga – can offer a taste of freedom. Some, such as drugs and alcohol, are more transitory than others. When they wear off, so does the sense of liberation they promised. It is often replaced by what I call a post-freedom hangover. Others run deeper. The taste of freedom they inspire us to move towards is slower in the making but it lasts longer. Every experience of freedom, whether temporary or long-lasting, brings in its wake a sense of our being released from imprisonment – our being able, even for a short time, to respond to life spontaneously with the whole of our being.

Bid for Freedom

Many, when beginning Cura Romana, have been struggling with their weight. They dislike – even hate – their body and suffer a sense of shame about themselves. These are heavy burdens to carry. Sometimes they labour under false beliefs about the impossibility of changing things. They can be plagued by frustration or anger. And, although seldom aware of it until it all begins to change on the programme, they also experience a deep disconnection between mind and body. Some feel imprisoned by cravings and addictions – not only to foods but to other things too, such as wine or cigarettes. They feel at the mercy of compulsions or unconscious habit patterns that undermine belief in themselves as autonomous human beings. They have forgotten that, like all of us, they have free will which enables them to make choices about what they will and will not do.

Probably the most freedom-restricting belief of all is the notion that what we want and need can be found only *outside* ourselves. It is a belief which, more than any other, prevents us from experiencing the depth and power of the essential being that enables each one of us to forge the life we want. It is time to set ourselves free from such constraints. Cura Romana begins the process. It is then up to us to take it further.

Unique to You

Freedom is a unique state of being. There is a boldness to it. You dare to say what you think and feel, yet you find it easy to listen to the words and hearts of others who think differently. It brings with it a sense of being able to trust yourself, as well as the Universe, even though you comprehend neither. It liberates you from the slavery of conforming to other people's rules, imprisoning ideologies, life-draining addiction and from the crippling influences of negative emotions that might have strangled you. The way in which authentic freedom blossoms for each of us is full of surprises. The freer we become, the more self-determining our lives become, and the more exciting. When big challenges arise, instead of appearing as crushing forces, they turn into worthy opponents. And wrestling with them helps us break through to an even wider experience of liberation.

In an outer way, to be free means to enjoy liberty of action under a government which is not despotic and does not encroach on individual human rights. In an inner way, to be free means becoming liberated from the relentless forces of doubt, self-criticism and fear that we all inherit growing up in emotional and educational environments that split our mind from our body and teach us not to trust ourselves. These environments teach us to put our faith in 'experts'; they neither teach us to honour the splendour of the individual human soul, nor do they tell us that the Universe is filled with compassion on which we can draw whenever we need support, and with power which we can direct to create whatever we want. Such freedom knows no age-barriers – no limitations. Neither is it the province of an elite few while the rest of us get by and hope that a few crumbs of this precious stuff will fall our way – if only we are patient enough, virtuous enough, or spend enough money buying the right products. Freedom is free. It belongs to all people – the demand for it is encoded in our genes. Perhaps this is what makes us long for it.

Breaking the Chains

The chains that prevent us from living in freedom are forged from our experiences – parental, religious and educational training, traumas big and small, and the *worldview* we carry, which acts as a filter to our perceptions of reality. Many still believe, for instance, that nothing exists outside material reality. Others are unconsciously driven by the false notion that they do not deserve to be free. Our political, educational and religious training almost never encourages us to listen to and honour our intuition or to trust gut feelings. Instead, we have been led to believe that it's better to turn to so-called experts for guidance in any matter – to follow received opinion. In the case of those who have long struggled with their weight, an important part of their worldview is the belief in much of the inaccurate information gleaned from the media. You have to exercise like mad to keep your weight down, for instance. You must exercise your willpower. Fat people should be looked down upon. Food cravings are emotional in origin and need controlling. The list is endless.

A worldview is a dominant way of looking at reality which remains unconscious in a culture but which tends to govern the judgements one makes, large or small. The prevailing worldview holds, first, that all phenomena in the Universe, even life itself, are nothing more than a complex yet ultimately explainable series of chemical and physical reactions; second, that differences between organic and non-organic life are only in degree; and finally, that the whole is nothing more than the sum of its parts. This mechanistic paradigm has been useful. It has enabled us to study and organize experience scientifically and it has been responsible for our technological development. However, the worldview on which it is based has blinded us to the breadth and depth of larger reality and made us feel like insignificant members of a mechanical and indifferent Universe.

Such assumptions have enslaved men and women throughout history, blocking our freedom, crushing creativity, limiting bliss and preventing us from receiving the gifts and grace of the Universe in all their beauty, wonderment and power.

Expand your worldview

Some of us climb to the top of the ladder only to discover that it was leaning against the wrong wall. Or we lose touch with our deepest dreams and longings. Instead of awakening each morning with that child's sense of wonder at what the day ahead might bring, we wake to a feeling of impossibility or regret. Perhaps we feel as though life is passing us by. Then, if we are fortunate enough, we realize one day that the rules by which we've been living our lives have not been our rules, but those we have unconsciously absorbed from outside sources. And we perceive an empty space inside – a gap that nothing seems to fill.

If this describes your experience, welcome. You've just entered the region of the soul. It's a wide, deep, uncharted terrain which many spend their lives trying to avoid. Yet so rich are the soul's gifts that nothing can take the place of journeying into the depths of yourself to claim the treasures buried there. Chronic fatigue, depression, loneliness and poor health are all calls from the soul. So are long-term struggles with weight and addictions, whether they are to coffee, drugs, alcohol, food or sex. They ask that we stop for a moment in the midst of day-to-day life and start to pay attention to the soul's whispers. Sooner or later this happens to everyone, even if they have come to a place of relative comfort in their lives, as I had. You have wonderful friends, a loving family and many blessings to celebrate. Ten years ago, without ever articulating it, I had come to feel this way. The life I was living was a good life – like a magic carpet on which I could ride. Would it not continue to keep me safe and content for ever?

Then something unexpected occurs – somebody dies, you lose your job, a marriage breaks up, flashes of long-forgotten memories surface, you get sick or badly injured. Suddenly our magic carpet is ripped from under us and we find ourselves tumbling through space. Fearful and confused, we wonder – with a strange detachment – if all this is going to kill us.

Welcome the challenge

Every challenge we face, all the hurdles and problems that arise, are calls from the core. They ask that we pay attention – turn within. They urge us to take up the challenge to connect more deeply with our essential being and learn to live our lives from there – by expanding through authentic freedom. They also pose an important question: can you begin to lay aside your self-criticism and limiting beliefs long enough to journey beneath the surface of who you think you are to find out who you really are? Homeopathic Cura Romana appears to open the doors of possibility of this discovery for those who want to use it as a means of transformation in areas of their lives beyond weightloss.

My own soul call – more a howl than a whisper – came eight years ago when a series of violent accidents rendered me unable to walk for more than eighteen months and prevented me from exercising for years. This plunged me into despondency, then culminated in another accident, which cracked my sacrum and rendered me immobile.

As it happened, my own soul's calls coincided with my having agreed to write a memoir about a traumatic childhood. I had been resisting the urgings of my longtime friend Gail Rebuck to do this.

'I could never write a memoir, Gail,' I said. 'I wouldn't know where to begin. Besides, if I were to tell the truth about my early life, nobody would believe it and the tabloid press might have a field day.'

'So what?' she replied. 'We live in a tabloid world. Look at it this way. That would only mean that more people read the book. Maybe some of their lives will be transformed by what you have lived out and learned to heal.'

After a lot of rumination, I agreed to write it. In constant pain from injuries, I retreated inside my walled garden to spend four years plunging the depths of myself as I wrote *Love Affair*.

Now is the time

What I gained by living through this difficult period continues to astound me. I discovered that, no matter how traumatic a life we have lived, no matter how many false beliefs we carry, no matter how distorted a worldview we have inherited, life-changing transformation can happen. And it can begin right here, right now, without the need for therapists, drugs or fancy programmes. Our body and our psyche have already been primed for it to happen.

For reasons I am only beginning to understand, the Protocol brings a realization of this to many. It seems to create for them an awareness that the power that fuels personal transformation is both universal and personal. How it happens is unique to each of us. Yet for everyone, it flows through us from the core of our being, fed by the universal energies in which each of us is immersed every moment of our lives. Recognized for its magnificence, and given half a chance, it begins with infinite wisdom and persistence to direct our lives while quietly dissolving chains that still bind us. Participants report that all sorts of false beliefs, traumas and pain rise to the surface to be acknowledged and released in much the way that physical wastes are on a cleansing diet.

It's important that we learn to look upon them when they appear – with a no-blame, no-gain attitude – as though we are watching through the neutral eye of a camera. Bless them when they show up. Each came into our lives to help us wake up, sometimes even to keep us safe, when we needed it. We do not need to know where they came from. But now is the time for us to let them know that we no longer need them, to bless them for whatever gifts they once brought us no matter how painful. Tell them they are free to return to whatever place in the Universe is their natural home.

So often, life's difficulties and disasters force us to create the time and space to sit in our skin and breathe softly. Gradually we learn to look upon our problems as bearers of gifts. As this happens, listening to the whispers from the soul becomes easier and easier. We realize they are there to guide us to the next step, and the next, and the next. And, so long as we are willing to let go of who we once believed we were, to discover who we really are, we gradually learn how to walk in freedom and live in bliss, regardless of what is happening all around us.

Freedom – the Real McCoy

Far too much vitality lies stillborn beneath patterns of addictive behaviour, fear and heavy psychological baggage – the kind of stuff we all carry around with us – to thwart our energy and make being who we are hard work. One of the most moving accounts I have ever read of discovering freedom came from a political dissenter imprisoned in a concentration camp in the early 1940s. He wrote about how he came to experience the true nature of freedom, creativity and wholeness while living in the most inhumane conditions of physical incarceration imaginable. He discovered his freedom in the only way any of us ever will – by coming to live from ever deeper layers of himself. Eventually, he wrote, the very soul of him and his outer personality became like echoes of each other.

The distortions we have carried – the false beliefs, destructive parental training, or negative habit patterns formed throughout our lives – gradually fall away. Rejuvenation begins to take place – emotionally, physically and spiritually – liberating life-energy and shifting the way we look upon reality, all the while allowing us just to be who we are. Pretensions or self-limiting assumptions no longer diminish the experience of being fully alive.

It's a Mystery

I have given a great deal of thought to why and how this homeopathic Protocol seems, so often, to initiate an expanded sense of possibility in many people's lives. Truthfully, I have no definitive answers. But I suspect that it has a lot to do with two things. The first is the intention with which you enter into and follow your programme. Some people are interested only in weightloss. Others tell me that they are at a point in their life where they feel themselves ripe for transforming on many different levels. Still others who do the programme for weightloss alone report that the Protocol itself has spurred in them a desire for expansion and spiritual deepening that they had not anticipated.

The other factor, which I suspect has a lot to do with the new-found sense of freedom that the programme engenders in many, has to do with the biochemical, physiological and energetic changes that take place in the body and the psyche as greater balance progressively occurs in the diencephalon. It's important to remember that the diencephalon lies at the core of the autonomic nervous system. As it functions better, so do sleep, one's sense of self and one's view of reality on many levels. Time to consider what you want from your programme. Like many who have gone before you, you may end up with more than you anticipated.

They say that each of us teaches what we most need to learn ourselves and creates what we most love. This is certainly the case with me and freedom. The most important thing I have learned from listening to my own longing for freedom is how essential it is that we learn to live from the core. The more we do, the more all living things are encouraged to do the same. I have also learned that when we become aware of the sea of powerful cosmic energies in which we are all immersed, it supports the journey towards greater freedom in ways that old Rousseau – despite his vast wisdom – could never have dreamed possible.

FEED ON BLISS

'FOLLOW YOUR BLISS,' the gypsy said. 'Connect with your inner light. Hear the sounds of birds. Taste the ocean's spray. Listen to the whispers of your soul. You were born to it. Bliss is your key to freedom. Have you forgotten this?'

The gypsy's words echoed in the woman's heart. She had never followed her bliss. She had always tried her best to do the 'right' thing, listened to the voices of others and valued their opinions above her own. She'd been on and off regimes, lost weight, gained weight, made money, spent money, found and lost lovers, taken part in self-help/self-improvement workshops and given up on them. Occasionally she felt she'd found an answer to something. Then it would melt away again like a long-forgotten dream. But that day, when she met the gypsy on the road, everything changed. The gypsy lady was old and wrinkled. Yet her eyes shone with a light so bright that the woman could hardly bear to look into them. What the hell, the woman thought, let's see what this old lady has to say. What have I got to lose? That was the day the woman let bliss into her life – that was the beginning of a journey of the senses that would transform her body and illuminate her life on every level.

Dive into Bliss

Bliss feeds your soul. It fuels transformation of body, mind and spirit. The human body is probably the finest resonator for bliss in the Universe. Why? Because a strong healthy body responds to every thought, feeling and sense perception it encounters. As human beings, we also have the distinction among animals – if we so choose – to be consciously aware of our responses. Throughout a million years of evolution, our DNA, connective tissue, emotions, energy fields, mind and power centres have been programmed for sensory awareness. Yet few of us have tapped our potentials for it. How do you hit the higher octaves of being? Dive into bliss. Then get ready to push the envelope of what you believed possible.

The emotional and spiritual transformations that take place on hCG+Food Plan begin as simple, physiological and functional shifts in the way the diencephalon area of the brain functions. The homeopathic – coupled with the Food Plan – acts upon the autonomic nervous system via the diencephalon. This does two things that give us greater access to bliss. First, it encourages the body to let go of toxic wastes which may have been held in its tissues for some time, rapidly decreasing the toxic burden a body has been carrying. As toxicity diminishes, our living matrix is enlivened and our senses heightened.

Second, the Protocol brings a calming, centring effect to the body, even quieting habitual thought patterns so that many internal conflicts and confusion are quelled. Physical illness often develops out of unresolved conflicts between our instinctual nature, which is centred in the diencephalon and other primitive parts of the brain, and the intellectual cerebral cortex, with which we are urged to govern our lives.

Simeons writes about this at length in *Man's Presumptuous Brain.*

> **Simeons says:** *An instinct is a very old impulse which is generated in the diencephalon by a combination of hormonal and sensory stimuli. In this process the cortex is involved only to the extent that it censors the raw incoming*

messages from the senses. An emotion, on the other hand, is the conscious or subconscious elaboration of a diencephalic instinct by the cortical processes of memory, association and reasoning. Emotions are thus generated in the cortex out of crude instincts. In primitive man many raw instincts were still consciously acceptable but in urban man this is no longer so. When a raw instinct . . . breaks through all cortical barriers, it is usually interpreted as insanity . . . raw instincts threaten the cortical authority with which man runs his artificial world.

Dangerous restriction

Simeons then goes on to describe the cortex as a censor of instinctual expression and action. Once the cortex changes instincts into emotion, it usually censors any expression of that emotion. And, because our culture is built on cortical control and it demeans instinct, illness occurs. As a result of these and other restrictions – both conscious and unconscious – directing our lives, we begin to lose touch with our bodies, our instincts and our bliss, and with our essential self at the core.

Our capacity for bliss, as well as our need to experience it, is inscribed on the primitive brain – almost as deeply as our need for air, water and food. Bliss is the medium through which mind, spirit and emotions weave a tapestry of meaning. Bliss renews. Bliss cleanses. It makes us feel whole, solid, stable and alive. Bliss tells us: 'This is something I want to try', then brings us the courage to go for it.

So important is bliss to becoming who we really are and to helping us realize our goals – whatever they may be – that when we deny our need for it, we are forced to look for artificial substitutes. Addictions arise: to food, drugs, alcohol, sex – even ambition. These addictions disempower us, leading us further from the authentic freedom that is our birthright.

Awaken your senses

Life is lived through our five senses. The more sensitive they are, the more we experience the multi-dimensional pleasures of every moment: the aroma of freshly made coffee, the touch of silk against our skin, soulful fingers on guitar strings, waves of orgasm to swell the body and silence the mind. The secret of employing bliss for transformation lies in becoming fully aware of everything you feel, touch, taste, smell, hear and see. Right here. Right now.

The Cura Romana programme takes you on a unique journey of discovery. A vital part of this journey is learning to make time for yourself, regardless of how busy a life you lead – time simply to be – to get to know who you truly are and to celebrate your life. Creating time for these things day by day, week by week, not only while you are on the programme but ever afterwards, automatically continues to expand your awareness. So does allowing yourself to indulge in the following practices, each of which expands consciousness:

Sounds matter Focus on a sound that pleases you. Let go of the world around you. This might be a piece of music, the sound of the wind in the trees or of birds at dawn, the flow of a fountain, the crash of waves.
Inner visions Close your eyes. Imagine yourself in a beautiful place where you feel at peace. See what comes. Intuitions? Mental pictures? Feelings?
Sight meditations Focus gently on a fascinating object – perhaps the flame of a candle, the petals of a flower, the swirl of water as it spirals down the bathroom sink. Become one with the object of your gaze. Notice how you feel.

Tune into your body

Without your body, without your ears and tongue, you cannot hear the voice of another, neither can you form words to express yourself. Without a nose, the delight of tuberose or vanilla will never be known. Without a brain, you cannot explore thought or dream dreams. Your body is far more than a vehicle for consciousness. It is consciousness itself – pure energy in crystallized form. The more blessed, the more loved, the more free your body is – regardless of its conflicting impulses and contradictions – to explore its place in the vast sea of energy that is life, the greater your creativity, your power and your capacity for bliss becomes.

As a culture we do not feel comfortable with our bodies. We often treat them like things separate from ourselves. As a result, they appear as dangerous shadows in films filled with gratuitous violence, brutal sex, and a misdirected lust for freedom at any cost to ourselves or others. Meanwhile, the exuberance of freedom, the joy of living in the body, the experience of ourselves as a radiant source of creativity and joy, continue to elude us.

What brings you joy?

Open your journal to a fresh page and begin to make a list of all the things that bring pleasure to your body or enliven your senses. Keep adding to your list as you think of more possibilities. Let your imagination run wild. At the beginning of each week, make a pact with yourself to enjoy one or more of these things within the next three days. Experiment. Find out just how much enjoyment your body can take! Your body thrives on bliss – feed it and it will reward you with energy, rejuvenation and joy that builds week by week into a whole new way of living.

Here are a few of my favourites:

1 Making love.
2 Running along the cliffs above the sea.
3 Smelling lilies and freesias, roses, jasmine and honeysuckle.
4 Watching a good movie.
5 Being massaged.
6 Dancing with abandon to wonderful wild music.
7 Feeling the breeze on my face on a bike ride.

8 Swimming naked.

9 Listening to all sorts of music.

10 Lounging in front of an open fire.

11 Reading a good book.

12 Spending time with a young child as they tell you about *their* stories and make-believe games.

13 Snuggling up to a favourite pet.

14 Eating fresh organic strawberries.

15 Walking in the rain.

What are yours? Write them down, then create an intention to make them a part of your life day by day.

Bliss asks us to immerse ourselves in a way of feeling and thinking, living and dreaming that can seem brand new. If you try some of the activities that bring you the greatest joy, you may rediscover ancient echoes of a way of living long forgotten. At the deepest levels, we have never forgotten at all. This experience feels like diving deep into a lake where the water is shot through with streams of light in constant motion – one moment gentle and lulling, the next wild or filled with the excitement of wind or the pounding of rain. This is what it is like for each of us as we come alive.

LISTEN TO THE
WHISPERS

CURA ROMANA HELPS liberate men and women from some of the relentless self-criticism, doubt and fear that we all accumulate growing up in a culture that splits mind from body and teaches us not to trust messages from within. It's interesting the way this appears to happen. It parallels the way that fat is shed.

As inessential fat deposits are burned up, turned into energy and lifted away to reveal more of the body's natural shape and size, what takes place to some on an emotional, spiritual, soul level – whatever you want to call it – mirrors the physical process. Distorting thought patterns and limiting assumptions, mistaken ideas about ourselves, which are untrue but which hamper us from living in the fulness of our being, often lessen and lift off. Thanks to the physical and emotional changes that take place on the programme, it becomes easier to listen to whispers from the core, to trust them and to act upon those that feel right.

Gifts of the Matrix

The more Cura Romana nurtures our living matrix, the clearer our consciousness matrix becomes. Step by step it is detoxified of false notions, fears and other people's rules. A genuine sense of personal value begins to develop. It then becomes easier than ever to hear whispers from the soul.

There are a number of simple practices which can be useful in encouraging this to happen: ways of writing, connecting with nature, playing with rest–work cycles, even of taking a fun walk to enliven perceptions. Each one can help you awaken to the intrinsic beauty of your essential being and come to honour it. All of them encourage you to become more aware of the magnificence of your physical body – something we so often ignore, neglect or vilify.

Come Alive

There is purpose and wisdom in the pulse of your blood, the flow of your breath, the flicker of your eye. Your body's power and influence, sensitivity and awareness, extend far beyond the limits of your skin. The living matrix – the whole of your being – is continually reaching out for transformation at every level. Moving through space and time it continuously changes. Cells die, others are born, as energies flow one way, then another, as the focus of your consciousness grows clearer. The paradox is that, through all this change, we retain our identity thanks to our innate essence which directs the process.

Universal Power

Our bodies are created out of the same light waves and particles that continue to shape the Universe we inhabit. We carry within us not only these energies but the Universe's power as well: a power to create from our intentions, to expand, to live in synergy with the rest of creation, to maintain balance and to transform ourselves again and again within one lifetime. In one sense, each of us *is* the Universe.

The driving force which animates our lives animates the cosmos.

Write Yourself to Freedom

One good technique for bridge-building between your essential core and your outer life is to write. The Cura Romana programme not only helps connect you with your physical body, but with your mind, feelings and aspirations as well. The physical act of writing freely whatever you feel or think, the good and the bad, can bring a sense of release, calm and clarity. Just let rip without judging anything. I don't mean sitting yourself down and making yourself do something 'virtuous' by forcing words down on paper. Far from it.

Years ago, wanting to learn how to write myself – by now, God knows, I've written millions of words, and am still learning – I read a book entitled *If You Want to Write* by a woman named Brenda Ueland. It inspired me. Ueland was a teacher of writing who worked primarily with people in slum areas in America in the 1940s. The book was published more than half a century before it came into my hands. She encouraged people to sit down with a pen or pencil and write truthfully whatever happened to come into their mind. In my opinion, Brenda Ueland is the finest teacher on writing in the English-speaking world, and she teaches nothing whatsoever about 'technique' (whatever that is). Her work has been much copied by others who have written books since then and who've made a lot of money at it. No one even comes close to her.

Guided by Ueland, I have seen people who sit down to write every single day, no matter what. They write whatever comes into their heads, it doesn't matter. They don't judge it, they just let it flow. The idea is, in letting it flow, you never take your pencil or pen from the paper. This is something that can't be done on a computer. It needs to be the physical contact of your hand from the pen or pencil to the paper. I have seen people's whole lives open up in a way that is quite remarkable by practising this.

It is a practice that I began a long time ago while thinking thoughts like: 'This is so stupid.' So what I did was sit down and write:

'This is really stupid, I can't believe that I'm spending time doing this every day.' I persisted. I never took my pen from the paper. I just kept writing. If I felt bad or angry, I wrote this down, always as specifically as I could. 'I feel terrible,' I'd write. 'I'm so disheartened, I'm depressed, I'll never be any better, the bloody birds outside my window are driving me crazy. I wish I lived in the city instead of the country where there weren't so many damned birds.' I wrote anything. It didn't matter at all.

I found that writing in this way creates an experience of bridge-building. Before long I noticed that some of the stuff that I'd been writing had become exciting. It was coming from some place in me that was not my intelligence and certainly not the part of me that often tries to 'do the right thing'. I began to enjoy the practice. I began to see that there was something in me I had never seen before.

I think this was probably the first time I connected with my own essential self. The more I wrote this way – by the way, the best writing I've ever done has been done this way – the happier I found myself. I rediscovered a tremendous enthusiasm, the kind kids have when they get up in the morning saying to themselves, 'Right, what am I going to do today?' Instead of: 'Oh my God, it's Monday, how am I going to get through till Friday?' – as 'responsible' adults often do.

I suggest that, on the way through your Cura Romana Journey, you might like to explore this practice for yourself. Sit down with a notebook, which only you will see, and begin to write. Write for 15 minutes each day – morning, evening, before you go to bed – whenever. If you wake in the middle of the night, this too is a wonderful time to write. Just let rip with whatever happens to come into your mind. Write as fast as you can in complete freedom, with no judgements of any kind. Do not go back and re-read or consider what you have written. Sometimes it can be interesting to revisit some of what you have written – but for now, just let the creative power at the core of your being flow through you on to the page.

The creative power within us works innocently. Like the thrust of being which comes from our essential self, it is quiet. It sees, it feels and it knows beyond our own conscious knowing. It lives in the now, in the present. As you allow yourself just to pour forth whatever words come, what you are actually doing is calling on your authentic being, coaxing it out and speaking to it – 'yes, yes, yes – let it happen.' Then you too are living in the present, spiritually, from the highest levels of your imagination. When you are writing in this way you are happy, truthful and free. There's a wonderful absorption that comes – very much like that of a child sitting in the middle of a room happily stringing beads.

What also develops out of your surrender to the flow is a sense of self-trust. This does not happen overnight. It can take weeks to sense it. Then, one day, as you begin your writing process, you know that something magical is happening.

Back to Nature

Nature is a carrier of sacred power. The energies of nature in which we have evolved for millions of years are *our* energies. Our own living matrix communicates holographically with that of plants and animals. At a cellular – even at a sub-molecular level – we *know* the familiar taste of herbs and smells of the earth. We are uplifted by the colours of a sunrise. This *knowing* and the pleasure that accompanies it are encoded in our DNA. Connecting with other living things expands our consciousness exponentially, fostering an ever-deepening connection with who we are. It also teaches us the skills enabling us to use the power of intentions literally to change material reality.

Mysterious Power

You can't hold your consciousness in your hand or draw a picture of it. Yet your own consciousness has enormous power to affect material reality. Researchers throughout the world have carried out well-designed multi-disciplinary research studies in what is often called the Human Consciousness Project. Their efforts converge to form a surprisingly coherent picture of the various states of consciousness available to us, and the rich experiences we can have as we begin to explore them. They have also discovered that blissful realms of expanded awareness – non-ordinary reality states – can be mapped just as we can map a country. Finally, consciousness research is demonstrating that entering *imaginal* realms (realms of awareness acccessed via mental images and the imagination) with a clear intention – such as listening to the whispers of your soul – when coupled with patience and compassion for yourself, can transform the world in which we live as well as help us manifest our dreams.

Claim Your Energy

Apart from permanent weightloss and greater vitality, what most people long for from Cura Romana is more energy. One of the best ways to experience it is to increase your awareness of your own natural rest–work cycles. Begin by listening to the needs of your body instead of trying to tell it what to do. Each of us has a different length of time during which we are able to sustain activity – either mental or physical – without losing interest or becoming fatigued. For most of us, these periods are much shorter than we think.

It's easier to judge tiredness from a physical activity than from a mental one because physical fatigue is more apparent. Yet mental and emotional efforts can be just as tiring as vigorous exercise or putting up shelves. It's no accident that office workers and women at home get treated far more often by doctors for fatigue than do labourers. If you want more energy, learn to become aware of when you are tired and develop the habit of resting instead of driving yourself even harder.

One way to check for fatigue is to notice which part of your body shows signs of it first. It could be your shoulders, your back or your eyes. It might show its presence in irritability or lack of concentration. Whenever your signs appear, heed them. Take a short rest. Even a 5-minute break will help you return to life or work with increased vigour and concentration. Tests show that people work far more productively when their work is interspersed with such breaks. The time spent on a break is more than made up for by the amount of time which would otherwise be wasted on unproductive thoughts and activities when you happen to be tired. When we continue to work although we are fatigued, the cells in some parts of our body do not receive the nutrients they need, nor are they able to eliminate wastes properly. They remain, as you do, at a low energy level. A short rest allows them to get rid of these wastes and take in some of the nutrients needed to revitalize.

The best break you can take when you need one is to do something as different as possible from the activity in which you've been engaged. If you've been working at a desk, for instance, get up, walk around, run to the corner and back again, splash cold water on your face. If you have been doing something physical, stop. Breathe deeply, then focus on something in the room for half a minute. It's a trick Buddhist monks know well. When you sit and watch a candle, a flower or a flickering light, you are released from that fatigued state where your mind and your body have taken on the characteristics of a dog chasing its tail. You slip into another mode of being, a more receptive rhythm so that your body can revive itself.

Free from the Core

Our longing for radiance – to live freely and fully from our core – calls us, asking us to expand our consciousness. It asks that we learn how to honour our five senses, as well as to move gradually beyond them, becoming multi-sensory beings. It asks that we reconnect with our instincts. Instinct, myth, dreams and metaphor are the 'language' of expanded realms. It asks that we come home to ourselves through them. We can learn to do this without drugs, without gurus, without becoming a disciple of anything or anybody, and without having to belong to any privileged group. You can do this regardless of age, physical condition or religious belief. The rewards are infinite.

Walk to Discover

While on Cura Romana, try walking in new ways and with a different rhythm. Just let your body move, and explore the new relationship to it that is beginning to develop. You may notice that former aches and pains are diminishing. This is a good time to begin letting go of a few of the worries you carry. We often think we need to make decisions about what we are going to do in the next hour, the next day, the next year. We worry about how to discipline our bodies and a thousand other things. Let go of these concerns and enjoy the rhythm of your movements.

Once a day, regardless of the weather outside, and whenever it suits you, go out walking for the sheer *pleasure* of doing it. It can be enormous fun to walk in sunshine, but just as wonderful to walk in rain – unhurried and unburdened by the need to 'look good'. Allow yourself to look around, to smell the air, to notice the way your body is beginning to move. Is it changing?

This probably sounds weird, but I do this often: when you see a tree, say silently to yourself, 'Tree.' When you see a flower – 'Flower.' This simple practice helps us become aware of where we are in space and time in a wonderful, spontaneous, improvising way. As we walk, life takes on an unexpected, exciting feel, while some of those futile internal monologues begin to fade away.

One of my favourite books was written by a musician named Stephen Nachmanovitch. It is called *Free Play: Improvisation in Life and Art*. It's a superb book. If you are interested in creativity on any level, and I don't mean just being an artist, but any kind of creativity, I highly recommend it.

In a chapter called 'Inspiration and Time Flow', Nachmanovitch describes a way of walking which I'd like to pass on to you. Of course, you are probably unlikely to be walking down a street in a foreign city as he describes, but much of what he writes about this way of walking is relevant. It reminds us that it is not impossible to live our lives moment to moment with real consciousness, real awareness and joy. He says:

A walk, following your intuitive promptings down the streets of a foreign city, holds rewards far beyond a planned tour of the tried and tested. Such a walk is totally different from random drifting.

Leaving your eyes and ears wide open, you allow your likes and dislikes, your conscious and unconscious desires and irritations, your irrational hunches to guide you whenever there is a choice of turning right or left. You cut a path through a city that's yours alone. This brings you face to face with surprises that are destined for you alone. You might discover conversations and friendships, meetings with remarkable people. When you travel in this way, when you walk in this way, you are free. There are no 'have tos' and 'shoulds'. You are structured at first only by the date of the plane departure. As the pattern of people and places unfolds, the trip, like an improvised piece of music, reveals its own inner structure and rhythm. Thus do you set the stage for fateful encounters.

I'd like to add that some of the 'fateful encounters' he speaks of are likely to be encounters with yourself.

Become What You Are

Transformation is at the heart of the Cura Romana Journey. Caterpillar into butterfly, base metal into gold – so life becomes an expression of who you are at the deepest levels of your being. Remember that, when it comes to personal transformation, experiencing dissatisfaction – even misery – can be a genuine blessing. It often fuels the process of transformation. Suffering can bring us to the point where we know something is missing in our life and make us ripe for positive change. Difficulties can awaken a desire to realize our highest potentials.

STILL POINT

E VERY CREATURE KNOWS how to be still. Cats laze in the sun. A furry caterpillar dozes on a tomato plant. The bumble bee nestles between two blades of grass. Yet we humans seem to be continually on the run. We have become programmed by the media, advertising and personal growth gurus to do it better and faster, to be more efficient, to keep going no matter what. We have lost the art of silence and still-ness. As a consequence, we miss out on the gifts that come to us when we are being instead of continually doing.

Stress Balance

Cura Romana offers you an ideal opportunity to rediscover the lost art of energy balancing. Participants begin to experience this as a result of the biochemical and neurological diencephalic improvement within the autonomic nervous system. As they progress on the programme, many find that handling stress – which used to be difficult – becomes progressively easier. This is quite a gift. Yet, like any boon, it's impor-tant that we reinforce the gift by coming to a better understanding of the nature of stress itself and learning what being able to move from a dynamic state of being into a receptive one at will does for lasting health and vitality. A simple practice we will be exploring later on in this chapter is an ideal way to do this. For the moment, let's take a quick glance at stress itself.

'What goes up must come down.' These words should be engraved on the brain – particularly of those of us who live full and busy lives. When stress gets out of hand it wears you down, creates the deep fatigue that makes you reach for coffee or sweets in a bid for more energy. When stress is prolonged, it makes you feel overwhelmed, destroys peace of mind and creates adrenal exhaustion to undermine health. Yet when stress is balanced by relaxation, it becomes the spice of life, excitement, the 'high' of living with heavy demands, knowing you can meet them and enjoy the process.

The autonomic nervous system – read diencephalon – not only governs your appetite, weight control, breathing, hormonal balance, sleep and sexuality, it also determines how well you deal with stress. As greater balance is brought to diencephalic functions on Cura Romana, it gets easier and easier to move at will from the dynamic high-energy stressed state into a deeply quiet, rewarding, restorative one. This is fundamental to ongoing energy.

Listen to the Rhythms

Every living being has two fundamental modes – solar and lunar. Physiologically, the solar – stressed – mode is the dynamic outpouring of energy and spirit. In the Orient this is called the yang rhythm. It is governed by the sympathetic branch of our autonomic nervous system. In its highly active state we experience excitement, the thrill of the challenge, the determination to make things happen.

The lunar mode, the yin rhythm, is its exact opposite. When lunar energy predominates we experience deep relaxation and restoration of body and psyche. Now the parasympathetic branch of our autonomic nervous system comes into its own. Instead of an outpouring of spirit and energy, we become highly receptive, literally able to draw energy, strength and bliss the way a cat does lying in front of a winter fire.

These two rhythms are like the sun and the moon. We need both to stay healthy and to provide ourselves with what I call rhinoceros energy – the kind of vitality that simply goes on and on. I learned a lot from watching rhinos in the African bush. Like all wild animals, they never waste themselves in unnecessary effort. Yet when you watch one run, its vitality sustains it with no apparent effort until it is ready to become still again.

A major complaint people make before beginning the programme is lack of energy. Either they tell of being trapped in the dynamic stressed state, unable to let go and calm their mind, or they complain of burn-out and have come to rely on stimulants from outside in the form of endless cups of coffee, sugar or drugs just to keep going. Unlike our creature friends, who instinctively know how to move from a dynamic state to a still point and back again, most of us have lost the knack and need to re-learn it so that it becomes second nature again.

Give and Receive Energy

When in dynamic mode, we are acting upon the Universe to make things happen in the world around us. When in receptive mode we are not acting upon anything. We are allowing the Universe to present us with many gifts through no effort of our own – you might say through an act of grace. I am reminded of the story of Martha and Mary in the Bible. Most of us are pretty good at being 'Marthas', but often we have forgotten how to be 'Marys'. The story goes like this:

Jesus stopped at Martha's home to visit. Mary was there too. Both sisters were delighted to see him. Martha went right to work, preparing food and cleaning. She wanted everything to be perfect. While Martha worked, Mary sat at Jesus' feet, listening. His words were like cool, pure water to her. She blissfully drank them in, not wanting to miss a single thing he said. When Martha noticed how Mary was sitting with him instead of helping her, she grew angry. 'See how Mary just sits while I do all the work. Tell her to help me,' she complained. 'Martha, Martha,' he said calmly, 'you're bothered by so many little things. Do you not know what is really necessary?' She looked at him with a puzzled face. 'It is Mary who made the right choice,' said Jesus. 'And it won't be taken from her.'

Few of us are ever taught about the importance of being able to move with ease back and forth from dynamic mode to receptive mode. As a consequence, our bodies are seldom at rest. Our minds are always busy. We don't know how to let go of endless internal monologues and troublesome thoughts. Forever thinking about the past and the future, we miss out on the creative joy of moment-to-moment awareness. We eat food but we don't taste it. We make love then wonder why it is not always as satisfying as we know it could be. We have forgotten how to live in the moment from the core of our being and let life flow through us instead of attempting to 'manage' it. In short, we have lost connection with the two rhythms on which lasting health, vitality and joy depend. Let's now look at the simplest and most efficient way of reconnecting with both – *zazen*.

Blissful and Vital

A powerful technique for re-establishing life-giving balance, zazen is a simple, yet almost infinitely transformative practice. I have used it a lot with Cura Romana participants, many of whom sing its praises and continue to practise it long after the programme has finished. In the process, zazen also deepens our connection with the innate self by simply becoming aware of the breath. Practise it daily. It silences the endless internal chatter, releases anxieties that stifle creativity and clears away internal monologues where our mind chases its tail like an obsessive dog yet gets nowhere. Zazen teaches us how to live life moment by moment. It trains the body and mind to be able to move at will from the dynamic, solar, stressed state into the deeply receptive, restorative lunar one the way animals can. This, in turn, strengthens vitality and teaches us the art of being present in the eternal *now* like a child, a sage, an artist, a lover.

Zazen has been practised for 2,500 years. It travelled from India, China and Japan to arrive in the West around the middle of the last century. The practice of zazen is neither a means of introspection nor of contemplation. It is a means by which we come to experience the unity with our selves and the Universe. As a technique, it is easy to learn and simple to practise. As with most valuable techniques, what matters is not trying to understand it, for there is nothing in it to be understood. What matters is doing it. As you do it day by day, it transforms your health and your life.

In essence, the human mind is meant to be like the still water of a lake at dawn. But, when the rains fall or the winds blow, its natural glass-like surface, which is meant to reflect the sun and the moon, gets disturbed with eddies and waves, distorting our perception of our bodies, ourselves and the world around us. As we practise zazen, our mind returns to its mirror-like state. Then it can reflect the world around us without becoming obstructed or distorted by anything in it. In time, we learn that we do not have to hold on to anything to create the life for which we long. We become free. This experience of freedom becomes contagious – a blessing not only for ourselves but for others. Marianne Williamson said it well: 'As we are liberated from our own fear, our presence automatically liberates others.'

Secrets of the breath

The word 'spirit' means breath – that is, life force. In Japanese they call it *ki*, in Chinese *chi*. In English we refer to it as energy or power. It is the electrical energy that fuels the living matrix of your body. Practice zazen and you learn how closely the way your breath is connected with the kind of thoughts you have and the emotions you feel. Working with the breath, you inadvertently work with body and mind. For these three are different aspects of a single reality.

As we develop awareness of the breath, as it enters and leaves our body, and of all the sensations this brings, we come to touch the still point and gradually develop a natural ability to focus the mind. We start by sitting in a comfortable but straight posture and counting the breath: inhale . . . 'one', exhale . . . 'two', and so on up to ten. Then we begin again back at 'one'. The point of the counting has nothing to do with trying to get to ten – it is just a simple tool. If you lose count and your mind begins to wander, notice this, bless your thoughts, whatever they are, then let them go by gently returning your concentration to the breath and starting again at 'one'. Each time you choose consciously to let a thought go and bring yourself back to your breathing, you increase your ability to place your mind where you want it to be. This is an incredibly powerful experience. After a while, you break free of the limiting thoughts, worries and obsessions that rule most people's lives.

Your sense of connection with your innate being grows stronger, as does your capacity to experience bliss, pleasure and the sense that you have the right to be who you are without having to conform to other people's imperatives. Your spiritual power grows, as do your intuitive skills. Creativity, which is closely woven into intuition, blossoms. We lose the sense of isolation which so many have where we feel alone and alienated from the Universe.

So let's get started.

Zazen

Position your body The way you hold your body – your posture – helps create your state of consciousness. There are many choices. You can sit tailor-fashion on the floor, using a small firm pillow, or zafu, which raises your bottom slightly off the floor. Sit on the front third of your zafu, tipping the body slightly forward. This creates the strongest feeling of stability. You can also use a chair. When sitting on a chair it is important also to use a cushion so that you can sit on the front third of the cushion and keep your back away from its back. Make sure your feet are flat on the floor. However you choose to sit, your back needs to be straight. Imagine that your head is pressing against the ceiling. Now allow your muscles to soften so that the natural curve of the back appears and the abdomen pushes slightly forward so that the diaphragm moves freely – rising and falling with each breath.

Position your hands Place your hands in what is known as a cosmic mudra, where your active hand (right if you are right-handed, left if you are left-handed) lies palm up in your lap. Nestle the other hand gently on to the palm of the active hand so that the knuckles overlap and your thumb tips just touch, forming a kind of oval. This connects your body's right and left energy fields. It also acts as a symbol for the unity of the breath, your life and the Universe. This also helps turn you inwards, away from the confusion and chaos of daily life.

Grow quiet Allow your body to settle into a comfortable posture. Your back is erect but never stiff, your chin is tucked in slightly, the tip of your tongue rests easily against the roof of your mouth, just behind your upper teeth, which keeps you from salivating too much. Breathe through your nose. Lower your eyes so that you are looking at the ground 2 or 3 feet in front of you. After a while you may be surprised to find that, although your eyes are open, you are no longer 'seeing' what you are looking at, since the focus of your attention will have shifted within.

Discover your centre This is the *hara* – the physical and spiritual centre of the body. It is a place of power from which all the martial arts are performed. Located in the pelvis, 2 1/2–3 inches below the navel, it is also the centre of gravity in the body. Allowing your focus of attention to rest at the *hara* creates a sense of balance for body and mind. As you breathe in, imagine your breath going down to the *hara*, then returning from the *hara* as you breathe out. Of course, on a physical level the breath is really filling the lungs, but imagining this helps centre you.

Breathe easy Pay attention to your breath without trying to change anything. Be aware of the tactile feelings that come with breathing. Notice the cool air entering your body as you inhale through your nose and what it feels like as it travels down the back of your throat. Feel the warmth of the out-breath as you exhale. When you stay in touch with this tactile sensation of breathing, you are less likely to be distracted by thoughts.

Count the ins and outs Inhalation is 'one'. Exhalation is 'two'. Inhalation is 'three' and so on until you get to ten. Then start all over again. The simple agreement you make with yourself is only that when the mind begins to distract you, you notice this and consciously choose to let it go, then go back to watching the breath and begin counting again from one.

Still-point practice

Zazen is as simple as that. Practising it for 15 minutes twice a day – preferably at the beginning of the day and the end of the day – we touch the still point within us again and again. In the process we begin to build up *joriki* – the power of focus and concentration so that, in time, instead of becoming caught up in the endless mental machinations that draw us away from living our lives fully whatever we are doing, we become able to choose consciously to let go and turn our mind towards whatever we wish. The connection with our innate being strengthens so that our inner world and our day-to-day life come together in harmony. The more you practise, the easier it becomes eventually, at will, to move into your still point even in highly stressful situations that once had you frantic.

Practising zazen day after day brings many other gifts from the Universe as well. Like the Cura Romana Journey itself, the practice of zazen is highly experiential. Trying to understand or rationalize either of them is a waste of time. Like most transformative practices, they will never be fully understood. Like Cura Romana itself, zazen can only be lived.

SHEER RADIANCE

Your Cura Romana Journey may be coming to an end, but this is only the beginning as your essential self continues to emerge.

Transformation is one of life's great mysteries. It is by no means easy. It demands that, like a snake, we be willing to shed skins when they become too small to contain us as we grow. Sometimes this is not an easy thing to do. For a time it can leave us vulnerable until a new skin grows firm and strong enough that we feel protected again.

Yet transformation is so exciting and so rewarding that who cares if you have to experience a headache while your body is detoxifying, or shed tears over the loss of a relationship. Such events are milestones along the road each one of us travels towards wholeness, authenticity and freedom – momentary experiences anchored in space and time, like sights we see while looking through the windows of a train on the most exciting journey any of us ever takes: the journey of our own unfolding within the magnificent web of life to which we belong.

Expanding the Matrix

Leading-edge research has amassed evidence that we are linked through our consciousness via complex energetic interfaces with other living organisms and the planet itself. This is the larger matrix to which we belong. Becoming aware of these interfaces, which are now being mapped by brain researchers, biologists and high-level physicists, can be fascinating.

Throughout ancient history, the basic unity of mind and body formed an integral aspect of man's belief systems and healing practices – from ancient Egyptian medicine and Ayurvedic medicine (the oldest known system of healing in the world) to Chinese medicine, shamanism and spiritual healing. Then, from the time of Copernicus and his heliocentric model of the Universe, this began to change. During the eighteenth century, and especially when the industrial revolution arrived, the awareness of mind and body unity was replaced by a world that stripped the Universe of soul, replacing it with a blend of mechanism and egotism.

Blinkered Horses and Mechanists

Our mechanistic worldview, which has developed since Newton decided the world was nothing more than a big machine, insists that:

- Mind is a function of the physical brain. It has no existence apart from the body and no power to create material reality.
- Intentions, prayers and dreams cannot change the material world.
- The only way we can gain knowledge is through the intellect.
- Phenomena such as ESP, out-of-body and near-death experiences are figments of people's imagination.

The Universe can be reduced to nothing but an accidental collection of material particles with no purpose and no meaning.

Not only does this worldview – now outdated – deny everything we instinctively know to be true, it contradicts every leading-edge scientific discovery made in the last hundred years.

Shifting Paradigms

No matter how useful any worldview seems, it has its limitations. Ours, for instance, led us to ignore the organic inter-relatedness of nature in favour of the notion that it is man's task, through science and technology, to 'harness nature' for his own ends. The mechanistic worldview also contributed to a sense of human alienation, expressed in our art and literature as well as in destructive social behaviour. As a result, what was once a dominant paradigm is exploding around us, thanks to discoveries in high-level physics, psychoneuroimmunology and the new biology.

Energetic links continue to be established between the inner and outer world of man. Complex interactions between consciousness and material reality are being mapped. The mechanistic worldview is on its way out. It is nowhere near big enough to explain the reality of now. As a result, new worldviews are rapidly evolving, some of which are playing leading roles in the development of authentic human freedom. Why? Because they help us break down the self-limiting barriers we grow up with.

Science Marries Soul

When people begin Cura Romana they often experience their body as something separate. Their minds are filled with the false idea that changing their weight and their lives can never be more than a dream. Then they learn otherwise. They discover just how connected it's possible to become on every level and how exciting it can be to live one's life in wholeness. As Cura Romana connects up body, mind and spirit in a harmonious way, you can begin to experience a natural lifting off and clearing away of limiting beliefs and false notions that have dogged you, bringing a new sense of self-respect and authentic freedom to your life. This process greatly clarifies and expands our experience of the world around us too. Every blinkered view of reality blocks freedom, entraps creativity, limits bliss and disconnects us, not only from our soul's blueprint and core nature, but from the Universe in all its beauty, wonderment and power for growth and transformation. The new expanding worldview is called *holism*. It looks upon the nature of the Universe as holographic. It was named after the work of scientists who demonstrated that living organisms are integrated energetic systems within an integrated Universe. Our brain and body are holographic. Each part of us, like each part of the Universe, is not only connected to the rest, but it embodies the nature of the whole within it.

The tension between the new holism and the old mechanism – which depended on a belief in separation between spirit and matter, form and substance – is important to resolve if we are to break out of the self-imposed prisons that limit our lives. We are being asked to let go of our preconceived notions about what's real in order to explore the further reaches of a wider, more exciting and transformative Universe.

Living Our Limitations

To be human is to live in a limited reality. It has to be limited to allow us to move about, act upon our environment and bring our visions into being. Were we continually to experience a sense of connection with multi-dimensional quantum consciousness, we probably would not have the drive to go about our daily lives. A few people whom I've met who seem to have this kind of connection often have little desire to go on living in a physical body.

Yet without a sense of connection to the majesty of transcendent realms, our lives become narrow to such a degree that we come to feel alone in an alien world. We don't experience the love we long for. We seem unable to create the things we desire. We feel ourselves not good enough, so we 'need' an expensive car, a new suit, a PhD to feel OK. If we get them we think they're great for a time. Then they too lose their

lustre and we our fascination with them. So we start wanting something else, continually caught up in a belief that 'if only . . .' everything
would be all right in our lives.

Gifts of Grace

Sometimes, when we fall in love perhaps, or when we are faced with
an event of life-shattering proportions like a critical illness or the death
of a loved one, a submerged area of our being erupts in magic, in
horror, or in surges of passion, energy and beauty. (Remarkably, as far
as death is concerned, again and again in the literature there are
reports that even in the midst of deep grief people experience a kind
of illumination which opens up a whole new world; they see life
afresh even when feeling the intense pain of parting.) For a time the
mundane quality of our everyday lives is replaced with a sense of
expanded being. We not only feel more alive, we wake up to find that
familiar things – the tree that stands outside a bedroom window, a cat
that greets us when we come home each day, the simple shell we
picked up and slipped into our pocket while walking on the beach –
have taken on a luminosity we can't explain.

Other times, without warning, while listening to music or walking
down a city street, we are hit with a sense that the world is far greater
than we ever imagine it to be, or a feeling that all we see around us –
in some way we can't explain – *is* us. We are all part of the same stuff.
While it lasts, everything seems right in the world.

Until now, to use Simeons' words, the presumptuous 'brain
people' have been determining the course of events in the world
through endless words and abstractions. Because the brain people are
not firmly connected to real life, they busy themselves with theories
and intellectual distractions that estrange them from their own
humanity. So great is their alienation that ultimately they destroy their
own lives, polluting the environment, destroying the forests, falsifying
the money supplies and trying to manipulate history to their own
ends. Ah yes, we say, but it is the brain people who took us to the
moon. Indeed they did. Cortical functions serve many wonderful

purposes: technology, investigation, and the development of stunning gadgets and ideas. But as Nobel laureate physicist Werner Heisenberg says, in modern physics thought has reached the limit of its usefulness. Now another sort of thinking is required.

Our belief in 'science' is dwindling rapidly as vast amounts of public funds continue to be spent to carry out inconsequential 'research', while simple, cost-effective solutions for health are completely ignored or are driven underground. As Heisenberg says, 'The violent reaction on the recent development of modern physics can only be understood when one realizes that here the foundations of physics have started moving; and that this motion has caused the feeling that the ground would be cut from science.' It is happening as we speak.

Western civilization developed out of a marvellous dynamism – a shining heroic impulse which crowns the spirit of Western thought. We see it in the gifts of Greek philosophy, the sculptures of Michelangelo, the music of Beethoven, the luminosity of the Copernican revolution – in moon landings, and spectacular cosmological images from the Hubble telescope.

But we in the West have also played the central part in creating an inexorable and multi-dimensional crisis on our planet: economic, intellectual, psychological, ecological, political and spiritual. To say the world has become dysfunctional is to beg the issue. We are already facing the possibility of massive catastrophe. For many life forms the catastrophe has already occurred. We look around the world today and sense that something is dying. We watch it, we feel it and we wonder what is going to happen next.

In the words of Richard Tarnas, author of *The Passion of the Western Mind* and *Cosmos and Psyche*:

> When it comes down to it, there is a spiritual crisis that pervades our world. I think it affects everybody, but the more informed and thoughtful a person is, the more aware they are of the reality of the spiritual crisis. We live in a world in which mainstream, conventional modern science has essentially voided the cosmos of all

intrinsic meaning and purpose. There is no spiritual dimension to it from its point of view. And yet human beings aspire to spiritual significance in the life they lead and in the world in which they live. It is only, I think, through going through a profound inner transformation, that one can see beyond that crisis and come into a world of a different kind.

New Beginnings

We stand poised at the beginning of a new millennium – a time of deep division and conflict, confusion and anxiety, during which much of what we have taken for granted seems as if it is being destroyed. This is also a time when we are being asked to let the old ways die in a healing process that will allow new ways of living, thinking and valuing life to take their place. It is a time during which, if we so choose, authentic freedom can be experienced for the first time by millions of people of all different races, creeds and colours. This can happen only if each of us is willing to deepen our access to wisdom, vision and compassion, both for ourselves and for the world around us. If we can learn to work and live in harmony with other life forms around us, we can use intention to create more balanced ways of living.

To bring such a world into being in a way that honours the highest potentials in ourselves, the animals and plants, rocks and sea, sun and sky, we will all need access to authentic power and authentic freedom. We will need to experience clarity of mind and compassion. And we must learn to use our freedom wisely. Such gifts do not come to us from *outside*. They will never be found in religious or political systems, philosophies or dogmas. The very best teachings may inspire us to open up our thinking in a way that sparks our own creative ideas and urges us to look more deeply within ourselves, to dream vaster dreams for our future and for the future of life itself. Wisdom lies not outside us in the words of politicians, bankers, scientists, doctors or philosophers, but within each unique individual soul.

Unique and Universal

Our uniqueness can be likened to the brushstroke a Zen painter uses to represent a shaft of bamboo or a leaf. What he paints is totally singular, like no other leaf that's ever existed. Yet within its uniqueness is encompassed universal beauty and life-energy of the highest order. So it is with each one of us as we live from our essential being. Within the individual genetic package which is you is found your very own brand of what I call 'seedpower' – a vitality that encompasses far greater physical, spiritual and creative potential than you could ever hope to realize in only one lifetime. The more fully your essential being is allowed to flow forth from the core of you, the richer your experience of authentic power and freedom becomes.

I once had an experience of pulling up a weed in my garden to discover that within its roots a marble had been crushed out of all recognition by the life force of the growing plant. So focused was the energy of spirit within the tiny plant as it grew towards the light, that nothing could stand in its way. So it is with the energy that animates us.

Amidst all the talk of shifting magnetic fields, galactic alignment, Mayan prophecies and economic upheaval, something life-transforming is being offered to each of us. It seems to be a process by which the light of individual spirit – unique to each of us, yet enigmatically universal at the same time – enters our cells, DNA and energy fields. When the light of spirit fuses with the density of the body, a flowering of our innate being takes place with unprecedented grace. Like the weed in my garden, nothing can stop it. It clears false beliefs that once held us back, enhances our health, heightens our creativity, expands our consciousness and fuels our capacity to live each moment from the core of our being for our benefit and the benefit of all.

RESOURCES

Because we live in such a rapidly changing world, the best source for up-to-date information on everything related to the programme is *www.curaromana.com*. There you'll find resources for the Protocol, which are continually updated by Leslie and participants. You'll also find inspirational reports from former participants, messages from Leslie and Aaron, the latest Cura Romana discoveries, links to video podcasts and much more.

Should you wish to embark on the programme, the website offers you two options. The Cura Romana Journey is a highly sophisticated day-by-day process including videos and audios to guide you from beginning to end. Cura Romana Elite is a personally mentored version of the Protocol in which you not only have access to the materials of the Journey, but are personally mentored by Leslie or a qualified former Cura Romana journeyer.

Here are the highlights:

The Cura Romana Journey

A unique online nine-week programme with step-by-step guidance to make this exacting Protocol work for you in the smoothest, most successful way possible.

What you get:

- Rapid Weightloss Manual.

- Consolidation Manual – Kenton's unique programme for lasting enhanced health and weightloss.
- 2 x 15ml bottles of our unique homeopathic.
- Daily guidance through each part of Cura Romana from beginning to end via Leslie's videos, audios and written materials.
- A personal online weight chart for monitoring your progress.
- Recipes and demonstrations from Leslie's home kitchen.
- Access to the online Sanctuary, where you can learn cutting-edge techniques to help you connect with your essential being, for greater freedom, creativity and joy.
- An extensive help section to answer all your questions.
- Online support when you need it.

Cura Romana Elite

The finest personal mentoring programme for transformative weightloss that you'll find anywhere. Your opportunity to experience one-to-one guidance and custom-tailored care each step of the way.

What you get:

- Everything in the Cura Romana Journey, PLUS
- Personal mentoring throughout your programme by Leslie and/or former Cura Romana journeyers trained by her
- Membership of Leslie's Inner Circle, giving you access to the latest discoveries and innovations for transformation of body, mind and spirit.

We are continually expanding our online programmes to make the Cura Romana experience more powerful, easier and more effective. Be sure to check in with us regularly at *www.curaromana.com*.

The Homeopathic Spray

We have deliberately restricted the outlets at which our homeopathic is available to ensure that the *back potencies,* from which the homeopathic has been formulated, are identical to the original source material from John Morgan. This is vital to the success of the programme on every level. There are four sources through which you can purchase genuine Leslie Kenton's Cura Romana® homeopathic. If you choose to order it online, it is shipped directly to you wherever you are in the world on receipt of your order:

- *www.amazon.co.uk*
- *www.CuraRomana.com*
- *www.Helios.co.uk*
- *www.Simillimum.co.nz*

You can also purchase Leslie Kenton's Cura Romana® homeopathic spray at the following stores:

Helios Homeopathic Pharmacy
8 New Row
Covent Garden
London WC2N 4LJ
England
Open Monday–Saturday, 9.30 a.m.–5.30 p.m. (local time)
Telephone: (44) 207 379 7434

Helios Homeopathy Ltd
97 Camden Road
Tunbridge Wells
Kent TN1 2QR
England
Open Monday–Saturday, 9.30 a.m.–5.30 p.m. (local time)
Telephone: (44) 1892 536393
Fax: (44) 1892 546850

Simillimum Pharmacy
20 Panama Street
Wellington 6011
New Zealand
Open Monday–Friday, 9.00 a.m.–5.30 p.m. (local time)
and Saturdays 1.00 a.m.–3.00 p.m. (local time)
Telephone: (64) 4 4999242
FREEPHONE within New Zealand: 0800 ARNICA (276422)
FREEPHONE from Australia: 1800 121795

RESEARCH INTO CURA ROMANA

Albrink, Margaret J., 'Chorionic Gonadotropin and Obesity?', *Am. J. Clinical Nutrition*, June 1969; 22:681–85. A negative review of the Gusman paper. *http://www.ajcn.org/cgi/reprint/22/6/681.pdf*

Asher, W. L., and Harper, Harold W., 'Effect of human chorionic gonadotrophin on weight loss, hunger, and feeling of well-being', *Am. J. Clinical Nutrition,* Feb. 1973; 26:211–18. A well-designed study yielding positive results for the Protocol. *http://www.ajcn.org/cgi/reprint/26/2/211.pdf*

Asher, W. L., and Harper, Harold W., 'Human chorionic gonadotropin treatment for obesity: a rebuttal', *Am. J. Clinical Nutrition*, May 1974; 27:450–55. Response to Hirsch and Van Itallie's objections to the analysis of their study. *http://www.ajcn.org/cgi/reprint/27/5/450.pdf*

Belluscio, Daniel O., MD, and Ripamonte, Leonore E., MD, 'Utility of an oral formulation of hCG for obesity treatment: A double-blind study'. Excellent photos showing changes in fat distribution on the Protocol. *http://indexmedico.com/obesity/hcg.htm*

Belluscio, Daniel O., MD, The hCG Obesity and Research Clinic in Argentina has been using a sublingual formula with over 8,000 patients. To see results: *http://www.hcgobesity.org/slideshow.htm*

Bradley, P., 'Human chorionic gonadotropin in weight reduction', *Am. J. Clinical Nutrition*, May 1977; 30:649–54. Letter to the Editor refuting the Stein study results. *http://www.ajcn.org/cgi/reprint/30/5/649.pdf*

Bradley, P., 'HCG clarification', *Am. J. Clinical Nutrition*, Jan. 1978; 31:3–4. *http://www.ajcn.org/cgi/reprint/55/2/538S.pdf*

Bray, G. A., 'Drug treatment of obesity', *Am. J. Clinical Nutrition*, Feb. 1992; 55:538S–44S. Mentions hCG negative studies in the Miscellaneous section. *http://www.ajcn.org/cgi/reprint/7/5/514.pdf*

Craig, Leela S., Ray, Ruth E., Waxlerm, Samuel H., and Madigan, Helen, 'Chorionic gonadotropin in the treatment of obese women', *Am. J. Clinical Nutrition*, March 1963; 12:230–34. A flawed study that did not follow Simeons' Protocol nor keep the calories to 500. *http://www.ajcn.org/cgi/reprint/12/3/230.pdf*

Frank, Barry W., 'The use of chorionic gonadotropin hormone in the treatment of obesity: A double-blind study', *Am. J. Clinical Nutrition*, March 1964; 14:133–36. A flawed study that used 1,030 calories instead of Simeons' Protocol. *http://www.ajcn.org/cgi/reprint/14/3/133.pdf*

Greenway, Frank L., MD, and Bray, George A., MD, 'Human chorionic gonadotropin (hCG) in the treatment of obesity – A critical assessment of the Simeons method', *Western Journal of Medicine*, Dec. 1977; 127:471. This study does not provide any information about the amount of hCG that was administered. Also, although the patients received instructions regarding diet and cosmetics, we don't know to what degree they complied with these instructions.

Gusman, Harry A., 'Chorionic gonadotropin in obesity: further clinical observations', *Am. J. Clinical Nutrition*, June 1969; 22:686–95. A highly informative and well-thought-out paper describing clinical work with hCG and obesity, including analysis of six studies which failed to reproduce good results with hCG. *http://www.ajcn.org/cgi/reprint/22/6/686.pdf*

Hirsch, Jules, and Van Itallie, Theodore E., 'The treatment of obesity', *Am. J. Clinical Nutrition*, Oct. 1973; 26:1039–41. A letter contradicting the Asher and Harper study results. *http://www.ajcn.org/cgi/reprint/26/10/1039.pdf*

Hutton, James H., 'The use of chorionic gonadotropin in the treatment of obesity', *Am. J. Clinical Nutrition*, Feb. 1965; 16:277. A letter to the Editor explaining why the Frank study failed to get good results and affirming good results using the original Protocol. *http://www.ajcn.org/cgi/reprint/16/2/277.pdf*

Hutton, James H., 'Chorionic gonadotropin and obesity', *Am. J. Clinical Nutrition*, March 1970; 23: 243–44. A letter to the Editor refuting the Albrink article. *http://www.ajcn.org/cgi/reprint/23/3/243-a.pdf*

Shetty, K. R., and Lalkhoff, R. K., 'Human chorionic gonadotropin (hCG) treatment of obesity', *Arch. Intern. Med.*, Feb. 1977; 137(2):151–55. This research abstract indicates that six women were placed on 500-calorie diets and that they were given 125 IU of hCG intramuscularly. However, it does not provide any information about the composition of the diet or any other important factors such as any medications that the women were taking. Considering that the authors claimed that hCG offers no advantage over calorie restriction in promoting weightloss, they presumably did not follow the Dr Simeons hCG Protocol accurately.

Simeons, A. T. W., 'Chorionic gonadotrophin in the treatment of obese women', *Am. J. Clinical Nutrition*, Sept. 1963; 13:197–98. Dr Simeons' rebuttal of the Craig study results. *http://www.ajcn.org/cgi/reprint/13/3/197-a.pdf*

Simeons, A. T. W., 'Chorionic gonadotrophin in the treatment of obesity', *Am. J. Clinical Nutrition*, Sept. 1964; 15:188–90. Dr Simeons' rebuttal of the Frank study results. *http://www.ajcn.org/cgi/reprint/15/3/188.pdf*

Simeons, A. T. W., 'The action of chorionic gonadotropin in the obese', *Lancet*, Nov. 1954, II:946–47.

Sohar, Ezra, 'A forty-day–550 calorie diet in the treatment of obese outpatients', *Am. J. Clinical Nutrition*, Sept. 1959; 7:514–18. Another failed study which did not follow Simeons' Protocol.

Stein, M. R., Julis, R. E., Peck, C. C., Hinshaw, W., Sawicki, J. E., and Deller, Jr., J. J., 'Ineffectiveness of human chorionic gonadotropin in weight reduction: A double-blind study' (Original Research Communications), *Am. J. Clinical Nutrition*, Sept. 1976; 29:940–48. An attempt to duplicate the Asher and Harper study that failed to do so. *http://www.ajcn.org/cgi/reprint/29/9/940.pdf*

Stein, M. R., Julis, R. E., Peck, C. C., Hinshaw, W., Sawicki, J. E., and Deller, Jr., J. J., 'HCG clarification: A reply', *Am. J. Clinical Nutrition*, Jan. 1978; 31:3–4.

Young, R. L., Fuchs, R. J., and Woltjen, M. J., 'Chorionic gonadotropin in weight control: A double-blind crossover study', *JAMA*, Nov. 29 1976; 236(22):2495–97. The research abstract does not provide any information about the composition or the calorie content of the diet, the amount of hCG used and the method of its administration. Considering that the study claimed that there was no statistically significant difference between those receiving hCG vs placebo during any phase of the study, the researchers presumably did not follow the hCG Protocol as it had been prescribed by Dr Simeons.

A link you might like to share with your doctor: *http://hcgobesity.org/ international_workshop/hcg_obesity_physiology.pdf*

Another successful study with before and after photos: *http://hcgobesity.org/research/Vogt_Belluscio_article.pdf*

Before and after photos from a successful clinical study on hCG: *http://indexmedico.com/english/obesity/hcgobengl.htm*

Other Research into hCG

HCG and Cancer Prevention/Treatment
http://www.foxnews.com/story/0,2933,153964,00.html

Human chorionic gonadotropin (HCG) induction of apoptosis in breast cancer *http://www.asco.org/portal/site/ASCO/menuitem.34d60f5624ba07fd506fe310 ee37a01d/?vgnext oid=76f8201eb61a7010VgnVCM100000ed730ad1RCRD&vmview=abst_detail_ view&confID=40 &index=y&abstractID=34924.* Scientists at the Massey Cancer Center at Virginia Commonwealth University confirming earlier laboratory research into the efficacy of human chorionic gonadotropin (hCG) in treating cancer. Using prostate cancer cell lines, hCG was shown to radiosensitize cancer cells as well as facilitate apoptosis, or normal cell death.

http://molpharm.aspetjournals.org/cgi/content/abstract/71/1/259
Prior work by Milkhaus Laboratory yielded positive results for breast cancer cell lines.

http://www.springerlink.com/content/e1wdnqd8g779phl7/.

Newsweek 4 Nov. 1996, 'AIDS' Achilles' heel?' (pregnancy hormone 'human chorionic gonadotropin' found to eliminate Kaposi's sarcoma) *http://www.encyclopedia.com/doc/1G1-18815782.html.*

http://www.encyclopedia.com/doc/1G1-19485292.html.

http://www.ralphmoss.com/gallo.html.

http://www.fccc.edu/news/2005/Pregnancy-Related-Hormone-hCG-04-19- 05.html.

http://www.breastcancertreatments.cn/?p=3.

http://www.wipo.int/pctdb/en/wo.jsp?wo=2000035469.

http://jcem.endojournals.org/cgi/content/full/86/11/5534.

*http://content.karger.com/ProdukteDB/produkte.asp?Aktion=ShowPDF&Produ
ktNr=224164&Ausgabe=228438&ArtikelNr=63378.*

http://www.obgyn.net/newsheadlines/womens_health-Breast_Cancer-
20040810-30.asp.
*http://query.nytimes.com/gst/fullpage.html?res=9B0DEFD81330F937A15753C
1A9609582608s*

http://www.patentstorm.us/patents/5877148-description.html.

http://www.freepatentsonline.com/5677275.html.

http://www.freepatentsonline.com/5997871.html.

http://breast-cancer-research.com/content/5/S1/31.

http://www.freepatentsonline.com/6805882.html.

http://www.thebody.com/content/art31492.html.

http://www.patentstorm.us/patents/6319504-description.html.

http://www.wipo.int/pctdb/en/wo.jsp?IA=US19970112028DISPLAY=DESC.

FURTHER READING

Allan, Christian B., and Lutz, Wolfgang, *Life Without Bread: How a Low Carbohydrate Diet Can Save Your Life*, Los Angeles, Keats Publishing, 2000.

Audette, R., *Neanderthal*, Dallas, Paleolithic Press, 1996.

Batmanghelidj, F., *Your Body's Many Cries for Water*, Falls Church, Virginia, Global Health Solutions, 1992.

Bertalanffy, L. von, *Problems of Life: An Evaluation of Modern Biological Thought*, New York, Harper Torchbook, 1980.

Bircher, R., 'A Turning Point in Nutritional Science', reprint from Lee Foundation for Nutritional Research, No. 80, Milwaukee, Wisconsin, undated.

Bircher, R. (ed.), *Way to Positive Health*, Erlenbach-Zurich, Bircher Benner Verlag, 1967.

Bohm, David, *Wholeness and the Implicate Order*, London, Routledge & Kegan Paul, 1980.

Burkitt, Denis, *Refined Carbohydrate Foods and Disease*, New York, Academic Press, 1975.

Challem, Jack, Burt, Berkson, MD, PhD, and Smith, Melissa Diane, *Syndrome X: The Complete Nutritional Programme to Prevent and Reverse Insulin Resistance*, New York, John Wiley & Sons, Inc., 2000.

Cleave, T. L., *The Saccharine Disease*, New Canaan, Connecticut, Keats Publishing, 1978.

Cordain, L., PhD, *The Paleo Diet*, New York, John Wiley & Sons Inc., 2002.

Crile, George, *The Phenomenon of Life*, New York, W. W. Norton, 1936.

Eaton S. B., Shostak, M., and Konner, M., *The Paleolithic Prescription*, New York, Harper & Row, 1988.

Fallon, Sally, Enig, Mary, PhD, and Connolly, Pat, *Nourishing Traditions*, Winona Lake, Indiana, New Trends Publishing, 1999.

Gittleman, Louise Ann, with Nunziato, Dina R., *Eat Fat, Lose Weight: How the Right Fats Can Make You Thin for Life*, Chicago, Keats Publishing, 1999.

Goettemoeller, Jeffrey, *Stevia Sweet Recipes. Sugar Free Naturally*, Bloomingdale, Illinois, Vital Health Publishing, 1998.

Gordon, K. D., 'Evolutionary perspectives on human diet', in *Nutritional Anthropology*, ed. F. E. Johnston, New York, Alan R. Liss, 1987.

Heinrich, Richard L., *Starch Madness: Paleolithic Nutrition for Today*, Nevada City, California, Blue Dolphin Publishing, 1999.

Kenton, L. and S., *The New Raw Energy*, London, Vermilion, 1995.

Kenton, Leslie, *Passage to Power*, London, Vermilion, 1996.

Kenton, Leslie, *The X Factor Diet*, London, Vermilion, 2002.

Kenton, Leslie, *Age Power*, London, Vermilion, 2002.

Kirkland, James, *Low-Carb Cooking with Stevia: The Naturally Sweet & Calorie-Free Herb*, Arlington, Texas, Crystal Health Publishing, 2000.

Kuhn, Thomas, *The Structure of Scientific Revolutions*, Chicago, University of Chicago Press, 1962.

Mackarness, R., *Eat Fat and Grow Slim*, Garden City, New York, Doubleday & Co., 1959.

McCullough, Fran, *The Low-Carb Cookbook*, New York, Hyperion, 1997.

Meyerowitz, S., *Sprouts: The Miracle Food*, Great Barrington, Mass., Sproutman Publications, 1999.

Morgenthaler, J., and Simms, M., *The Smart Guide to the Low-Carb Anti-Aging Diet*, Petaluma, California, Smart Publications, 2000.

Oschman, J. L., *Energy Medicine – The Scientific Basis of Bioenergy Therapies*, Salem, New Hampshire, Churchill Livingstone, 2000.

Price, W., *Nutrition and Physical Degeneration*, 6th ed., New Canaan, Connecticut, Keats Publishing Inc., 1997.

Sahelian, Ray, MD, and Gates, Donna, *The Stevia Cookbook: Cooking with Nature's Calorie-Free Sweetener*, New York, Avery, 1999.

Schrödinger, Erwin, *What is Life? and Mind and Matter?*, Cambridge, Cambridge University Press, 1980.

Simms, Mia, *The Smart Guide to Low-Carb Cooking*, Petaluma, California, Smart Publications, 2000.

Taubes, Gary, *Good Calories, Bad Calories – Challenging the Conventional*

Wisdom on Diet, Weight Control, and Disease, New York, Alfred Knopf, 2007.

Weil, Andrew, MD, *Spontaneous Healing: How to Discover and Enhance Your Body's Natural Ability to Maintain and Heal Itself*, New York, Ballantine Books, Random House Inc., 2000.

Zukav, G., *The Dancing Wu Li Masters*, New York, William Morrow, 1979.

BIBLIOGRAPHY

Angel, J. L., 'Health as a crucial factor in the changes from hunting to developed farming in the Eastern Mediterranean', in *Paleopathology at the Origins of Agriculture*, eds M. N. Cohen and G. J. Armelagos, New York, Academic Press, 1984.

Bower, B., 'The two million year old meat and marrow diet resurfaces', *Science News*, Jan. 1987, 3.

Carpenter, K. J., 'Protein requirements of adults from an evolutionary perspective', *Am. J. Clinical Nutrition*, 1992, 55.

Cassidy, C. M., 'Nutrition and health in agriculturalists and hunter-gatherers: A case study of two prehistoric populations', in *Nutritional Anthropology, Contemporary Approaches to Diet and Culture*, eds N. M. Jerome, R. F. Kandel and G. H. Felto, Pleasantville, New York, Redgrave Publishing Co., 1980.

Eaton, S .B., 'Humans, lipids and evolution', *Lipids*, 1992, 27.

Eaton, S. B. and Konner, M. J., 'Paleolithic Nutrition: A consideration of its nature and current implications', *New England J. Medicine*, 1985.

Eaton, S. B. et al., 'An evolutionary perspective enhances understanding of human nutritional requirements', *European J. Nutrition*, 1996, 126.

Eaton, S. B. et al., 'Stone agers in the fast lane: Chronic degenerative diseases in evolutionary perspective', *Am. J. Medicine*, 1988, 84.

Eaton, S. B., Eaton, S. B. III, and Konner, M. J., 'Paleolithic nutrition revisited: A twelve-year retrospective on its nature and implications', *European J. Clinical Nutrition*, 1997.

Foster, D. W., 'The Banting Lecture 1984: From glycogen to ketones – and back', *Diabetes*, 1984, 33.

Lieb, C. W., 'The effects of an exclusive, long-continued meat diet', *JAMA*, 1926, 87 (1).

Lieb, C. W., 'The effects on human beings of a twelve month exclusive meat diet', *JAMA*, 1929, 93 (1).

O'Dea, K., 'Glucose and insulin responses to carbohydrate ingestion: acute and long term consequences', *Obesity, Dietary Factors and Control*, ed. Rosmos et al., Tokyo, Japan Scientific Societies Press, 1991.

Oschman, J. L., 'Structure and properties of ground substances', *Am. Zoologist*, 1984, 24.

Pottenger, F. M. Jr, 'The Effect of Heat Processed Foods', *Am. J. Orthodontistry and Oral Surgery*, 1946, 32(8).

Torjeson, P. A., et al., 'Lifestyle changes may reverse development of insulin resistance syndrome', *Diabetes*, 1997, 20.

CONVERSION TABLES

Measurement Conversions

British	US	Metric
1 teaspoon	= 1 teaspoon	= 5 ml
1 dessertspoon	= 2 teaspoons	= 10 ml
1 tablespoon	= 1 tablespoon	= 15 ml
2 fluid ounces	= 1/4 cup	= 60 ml
4 fluid ounces	= 1/2 cup	= 120 ml
1 teacup	= 1 cup	= 240 ml
4/5 imperial pint	= 2 cups	= 480 ml
1 pound	= 1 pound	= 454 grams

Note: 1 US pint = 16 fluid ounces
1 imperial pint = 20 fluid ounces

US Cooking Measures

3 teaspoons	= 1 tablespoon	= 1 ounce
4 tablespoons	= 1/4 cup	= 2 ounces
1 stick butter	= 1/2 cup	= 4 ounces
2 cups	= 1 pint	= 1 pound
1 pint	= 16 ounces	= 1 pound
4 cups	= 1 quart	= 2 pounds

Oven Temperatures

Fahrenheit	Celsius	Heat	Gas No.
150	65	Warm	Pilot light
225	107	Very slow	1/4
250	121	Very slow	1/2
275	135	Very slow	1
300	149	Slow	2
325	163	Slow	3
350	177	Moderate	4
375	191	Moderate	5
400	204	Hot	6
425	218	Hot	7

ACKNOWLEDGEMENTS AND DEDICATION

So many people have helped me learn what I needed to know to write this book – from A. T. W. Simeons, whose brilliance and practical wisdom long inspired me, to my dear Bavarian doctor friend who introduced me to the programme all those years ago. I must also thank John Morgan, who generously worked with me to perfect the formulation of our unique homeopathic, and the many doctors in Europe, the United States and South America who have shared with me their own experiences of the Protocol.

Some wonderful friends and helpmates have made the writing of this book possible, including my daughter Susannah, who knows the Protocol backwards and forwards having experienced it twice herself; Jan Neeson, whose computer skills, intelligence and devotion to the project have been invaluable; and my son Aaron, who created *www.CuraRomana.com* and brings such conscientious care to all who are on the programme.

I am infinitely grateful to the Bantam Press team, who have given so much of their time, their creativity and dedication to this book, as I am to my dear friend Gail Rebuck for her belief in the importance of the project and her introduction to my editor, Brenda Kimber. Brenda possesses an extraordinary combination of brilliance, passion, dedication and warmth. Without these people the project would never have been born. My heartfelt thanks also go to Katrina Whone, Vivien Garrett, Brenda Updegraff, Phil Lord, Patsy Irwin, Elizabeth Swain, Sarah Whittaker and Elspeth Dougall. You guys are the best!

Above all, I want to thank each and every one of the hundreds of men and women who have trusted me to mentor them through their individual Cura Romana Journeys. Their honesty, courage and passion to explore what the Protocol has to offer have made this a wonderful journey for me too. To list them all would take up pages: you know who you are. I hope you also know how precious the time we have spent together has been for me. Thank you. It is to you and to others like you who have longed to bring their struggle with overweight to an end that this book is dedicated.

INDEX

meta-analysis study 51–2
metabolic reset 12–13, 16, 54, 60–3, 75,
    101–4, 113, 116, 186, 188, 193, 199,
    200, 202, 220, 278
    programme 16, 17–18
metabolic syndrome 52–3
metabolism, slowing 171
Mexican restaurants 280
Michelangelo Buonarotti 47–8
micro-filtered whey 60, 120, 121, 188,
    226, 234, 246, 279, 281
migraine headaches ix
milk products, and sensitivities 217
mineral oils rule 75–6
Monsanto 118
Morgan, John 13–14, 287
muesli, live 244–5
muscle mass, and Cura Romana 178

National Academy of Sciences report
    Diet and Health 27
National Institutes of Health, obesity
    outcome research 54
nature, connecting with 317
neo-apple days 282
neolithic humans, diet 29, 30–1
nervous system, fuel for 204–5
neurosis, hCG treatment 44
Newton, Sir Isaac 331
nutritional supplements 179, 189
nuts, and sensitivities 217

O'Rourke, P. J. 206
obesity
    as metabolic disorder 23–5, 27–8,
        36–47
    false assumptions 26–7, 35
    inherited 28–31, 38–9
    outcome research (NIH) 54
    pathology 45–7, 54–5
    Simeons and 21–5, 27–34
    studies 45–56
oils/ fats
    fats, avoidance, hCG+Food Plan
        114–16
    choosing, rules for 238–9
    skin absorption 4, 69, 74–6, 77–9,
        113, 115–16, 174

omega-3 group of fats 209–11
omega-6 group of fats 209–10
one-bowl meals 243
Onion Caramelized Shellfish 143
Orange and Fennel Salad 151
Orange Frappe 169
Orange Zest 260
organic foods 113, 114, 116, 117, 121–5,
    127, 188, 233, 234, 236, 245
Oschman, James L., *Energy Medicine –
    The Scientific Basis* 275
osteopenia, hCG treatment 45
over-enthusiasm, and Consolidation 187

Palaeolithic diet 29–30, 203, 277
Pan-Seared Steak 145–6
pancakes 247–8
pesto 257
pie crust 272
pituitary gland, and obesity xi, 36
plateaux, handling 126–30, 174
postprandial thermogenesis 187–8
posture, and consciousness 327–8
Prawns Marinara 141
pregnancy
    hCG and 40, 41–3
pregnant women, weightloss 171
prehistoric diet 29–30, 203, 277
prescription medication, Cura Romana
    programme and 67–8
Price, Weston, *Nutrition and Physical
    Degeneration* 196
prostaglandin 208, 209, 210
protein dishes, Consolidation 264–6
protein foods
    Consolidation 229–30, 187–9
    hCG+Food Plan 111
protein/green powder mix 281
Protocol, following 59–61, 68–71, 82–8,
    90–1
psychoses, hCG treatment 45
psyllium (*Plantago asiatica*) 73, 76, 109,
    227, 246
Pub Med database 50
puberty, and Cura Romana 181

questions answered, hCG+Food Plan
    170–82

NOTES

ABOUT THE AUTHOR

Award-winning writer, television broadcaster and teacher, Leslie Kenton is well known in the English-speaking world for her no-nonsense, in-depth reporting. According to London's *Time Out*, 'If there is one health expert who can genuinely be described as pioneering and visionary, it is Leslie Kenton.' Her network television series include *Raw Energy, Ageless Ageing* and the *To Age or Not To Age* documentary that made television history when the diet and exercise programme she designed reversed the parameters of ageing in medically measurable ways. She also conceived and created the world-wide Origins range for Estée Lauder. A former consultant to the European Parliament for the Green Party and course developer for Britain's Open University, Leslie has written more than thirty-five books on health, beauty and spirituality. Trained in acupuncture, nutrition, bioenergetics and energy medicine, Leslie is a member of AAMET and NTCB in the United States and a certified homeo-therapeutics consultant. In the UK, her contribution to natural health has been honoured by her having been asked to deliver the McCarrison Lecture at the Royal Society of Medicine. An American by birth, Leslie now divides her time between her homes in Primrose Hill, London and South Island, New Zealand. You can find out more about her work at *www.lesliekenton.com*, *www.curaromana.com* and *loveaffair-thebook.com*.